The Clean Eating Cookbook & Diet

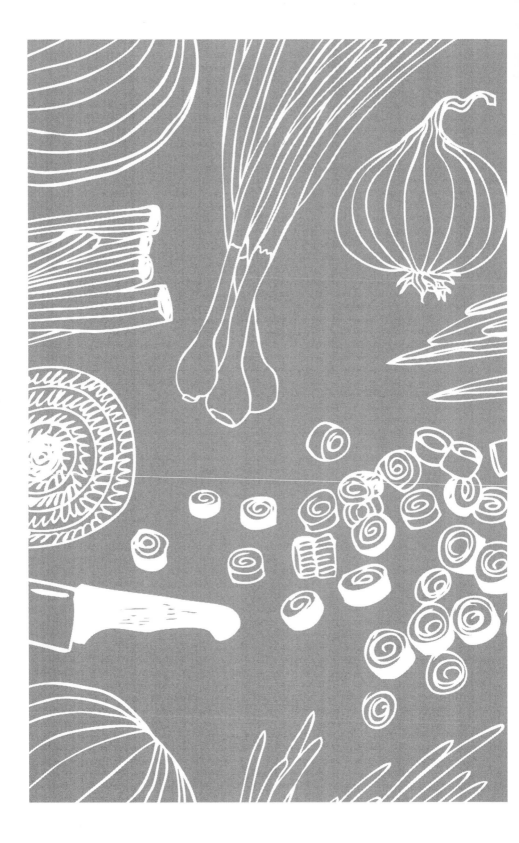

OVER **100** HEALTHY
WHOLE FOOD RECIPES
& MEAL PLANS

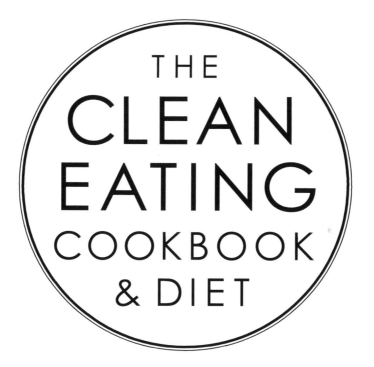

THE
CLEAN
EATING
COOKBOOK
& DIET

ROCKRIDGE
PRESS

Contents

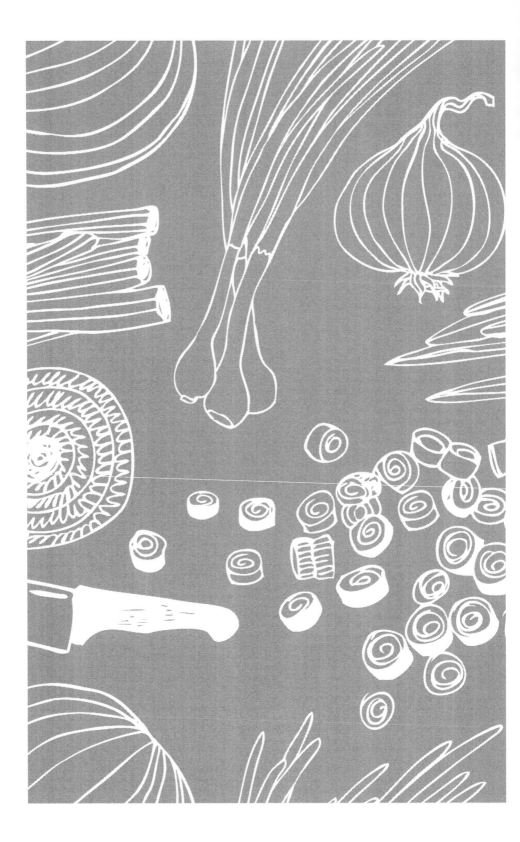

Introduction

Clean Eating isn't a new idea, but it's certainly one that's gaining popularity—because it works. It isn't a standard diet that you follow short-term to reach a single health or body goal; it's a lifestyle. On this plan, you won't be eliminating whole food groups or starving yourself, as these approaches aren't sustainable and do nothing but produce short-term weight loss. Clean Eating is about a lifetime of enjoying natural, unprocessed foods that taste good and nourish you, paving the way to a stronger, fitter body.

To help you better understand Clean Eating, this book is arranged in an easy-to-follow format that will show you the why, what, and how of this healthful lifestyle.

The Clean Eating Cookbook & Diet offers a path to a healthful lifestyle with:

- A thorough explanation of what Clean Eating is and how it evolved, along with the benefits of embracing this lifestyle
- A season-by-season outline of what to eat and when, what foods to avoid, and "super foods" that you should include whenever possible in your meal plans
- The essentials of Clean Eating, including the importance of exercise, dos and don'ts of the plan, and some simple steps for getting started on the path to good health
- A two-week meal plan, complete with comprehensive shopping lists, that will give you a good idea about how Clean Eating works and will allow you to begin your journey immediately
- Important information about how to prepare and cook your Clean Eating foods once you bring them home from the supermarket. Knowing which cooking methods to use, becoming familiar with herbs and spices, and understanding your many whole-grain options are invaluable when eating cleanly
- 105 Clean Eating recipes to get you started on the right foot

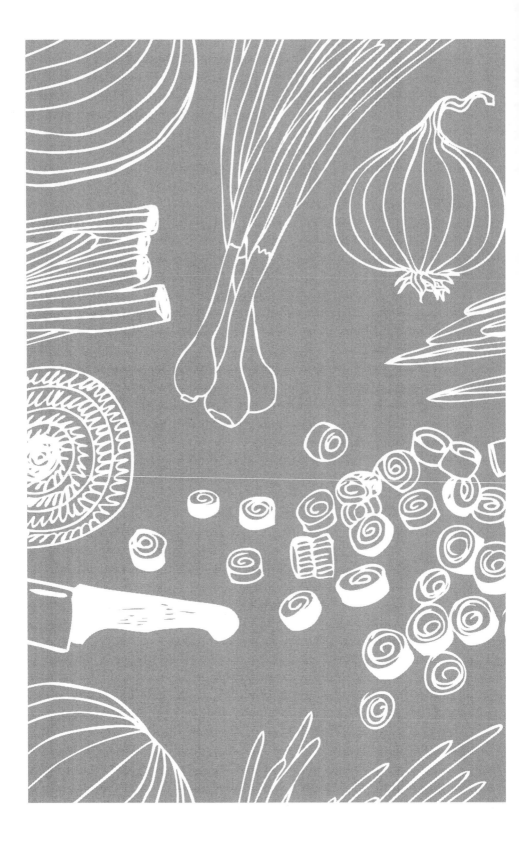

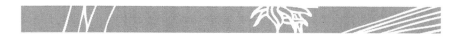

PART ONE

Fundamentals of Clean Eating

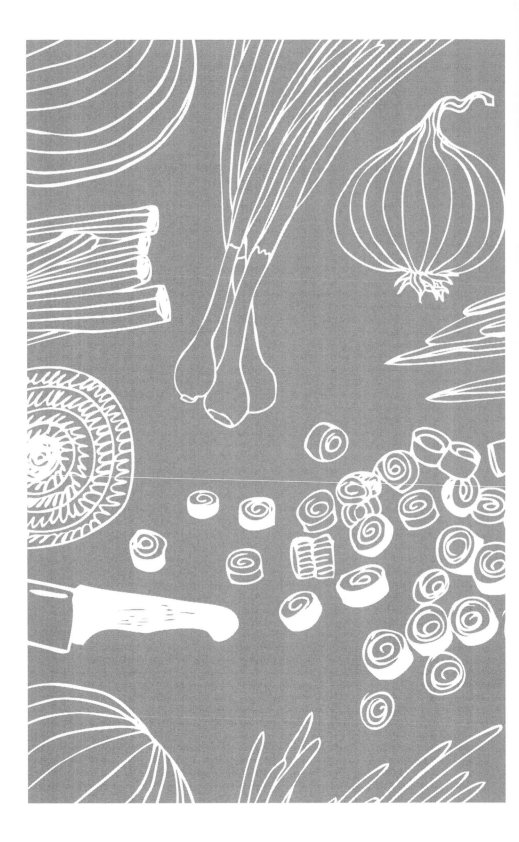

CHAPTER ONE

Clean Eating Principles

Do you sometimes feel like food controls you? Are you searching for a solution to your health or weight issues? Do you exercise but don't see the results you want in the mirror, and still don't feel energetic and healthy? Have you counted calories, cut out carbohydrates and fats, and shaken up countless smoothies in the quest for better health?

Clean Eating might be the solution for you if you're ready for a lifestyle change that will help you get in the healthiest shape of your life. You'll eat delicious meals without feeling hungry or deprived, and you'll enjoy the benefits of caring for yourself with nutritious whole food.

WHAT IS CLEAN EATING?

So what exactly is Clean Eating, and how is it different from every other eating plan out there?

Clean Eating isn't like diets you might have tried that keep your calories at starvation levels, exclude entire food groups, and require you to live on supplements. It's a way of eating that's sustainable over your entire life and will let you enjoy peak health while savoring delicious food.

In a nutshell, Clean Eating is about choosing foods that are as close to their natural state as possible. For example, strawberries are natural, but strawberry jam isn't. While following the plan, you'll cut out processed foods of any kind, such as sugar, refined grain, and saturated fats, and replace them with fruits, vegetables, lean protein, whole grains, and good fats. You'll eat small meals five to six times a day and exercise in moderation.

Eating cleanly will change the relationship you have with food. You'll come to understand that fueling your body with the kinds of food that it's meant to eat creates vibrant good health with no feelings of deprivation or fatigue. Clean

Eating is meant to be sustainable in the long term, so it's important to approach it from a practical standpoint. You won't be shooting for perfection in all of your choices, just a genuine commitment to better health and eating what nurtures and nourishes your body. You can certainly have a treat every once in a while, such as a piece of dark chocolate or even a small slice of birthday cake with friends. But after enjoying a bounty of healthful choices, you might find that sweets and salty snacks just aren't as tempting as they used to be.

THE HISTORY OF CLEAN EATING

Diets, and weight loss in particular, are big business, because even though scientific research points to food as the key to good health, people are getting fatter and weight-related chronic diseases are on the rise. There have been many strange fad diets on the health scene over the years—ones that promote eating only cabbage soup, grapefruit, or even fast food, for example. The concept of Clean Eating emerged as an alternative to these trendy nutrition disasters, and it has remained a logical choice for many people seeking a healthier life.

The concept of eating cleanly is definitely not new; it's only new on the popular radar. Many people never heard of Clean Eating before Tosca Reno, a Canadian fitness model, started promoting it in her line of popular books. The compelling story of her journey from frumpy housewife to sculpted health guru made Clean Eating sexy and exciting. Who wouldn't want to experience such a spectacular, positive life change?

Reno's Clean Eating book series catapulted the diet into the spotlight, but this healthful eating strategy actually has its roots in the 1960s and 1970s in the natural whole-foods revolution that promoted unprocessed (and ideally organic) foods. Chemically altered and processed foods proliferated in the supermarket aisles, and the natural food movement was born to oppose the "faux food" pushed by corporations. The Clean Eating philosophy of those who strove to eat natural foods started to make sense to more and more people when obesity rates began skyrocketing and weight-related diseases became widespread.

Seeking a healthier life for themselves and their families, an increasing number of consumers started rejecting processed foods, refined ingredients, sugar, saturated fats, and foods with little or no nutritional value. Clean Eating enthusiasts such as Tosca Reno have devised a simple, logical eating blueprint, and fans have embraced it with commitment and great success. Clean Eating isn't a fad diet; it's the simple concept of fueling your body with wholesome, nutritious foods.

THE EXPERTS' VIEW: SCIENCE AND RESEARCH

Although eating cleanly seems like a common sense strategy for a healthier, more energized lifestyle, there are people who criticize the concept or the essential rules of the plan. Some critics feel that it's impossible to eat cleanly because the food available today is intrinsically "unclean" even when pro-duced organically. This might be the case, but in the end, taking steps to eat mindfully—as realistically clean as possible—is what Clean Eating is all about. Experts can't dismiss the basic principles of Clean Eating because most of the current research on nutrition supports its strategies, at least in part. Almost without exception, nutrition and weight-loss experts endorse Clean Eating's central guidelines:

- **Eat small meals every two to three hours:** Eating cleanly at regular intervals cuts the risk of snacking because it keeps your blood sugar level from dropping too low. You have fewer cravings and less chance of binge eating on harmful foods (Hyman 2012). It's important to fit these small meals into your routine as conveniently as possible and to eat healthful foods whenever you're hungry. Use your best judgment.
- **Never skip a meal, and always carry Clean Eating foods with you:** This will help you maintain a stable blood sugar level and avoid snacking on the wrong foods (Hyman 2012). A hectic schedule can make it difficult to find wholesome food on the go, but bringing the bounty with you makes it easy to eat healthfully and stay the course.
- **Watch portion sizes:** Many people have no idea what a correct portion size looks like, and their perceptions are significantly distorted by the huge portions served in U.S. restaurants (WebMD 2012). The Clean Eating plan is based on good portion sizing rather than calorie-counting, giving you an effective way to control the amount of food you eat.
- **Consume good fats, limit saturated fats, and avoid trans fats:** Many diets completely exclude fat in all forms, which is a bad idea, because your body needs fat for many functions. In particular, it's crucial to take in essential fatty acids (see the glossary) since your body can't make them

on its own (Teicholz 2007). Eating good fats and avoiding bad fats will reduce your risk of cardiovascular disease.

- **Avoid processed foods, refined ingredients, and sugar:** This is sound advice because many of these products are empty-calorie, high-sodium, and fat-laden foods. Replacing processed foods with wholesome natural choices is the foundation of Clean Eating, and fuels your body with every bite.

Clean Eating is a well-rounded, balanced plan that doesn't exclude any food group or require you to use unfamiliar, hard-to-find ingredients. The emphasis is on vegetables, fruit, whole grains, lean protein, good fats, and lots of water. Eating cleanly can easily become a routine that you can follow comfortably for your whole life. The fact that this plan doesn't restrict calories is also a plus; countless people have wrecked their metabolism by suffering through starvation-style fad diets that did nothing for them in the long run (Tomiyama et al. 2010). Calories do still matter, of course—too many will create weight gain—but the *types* of food you eat are just as important. Clean foods fill you up, so you're less likely to snack on high-calorie foods.

When you pair exercise with Clean Eating, you help tip the scales further in the right direction. Exercise on a regular basis will help control your appetite and food cravings as well as burn calories and speed up your metabolism. Moving your body and weight training can also reduce stress, lower your blood pressure, and help prevent osteoporosis.

Clean Eating is based on common sense rather than science: it's only logical to limit your exposure to anything—including food—that can have a negative effect on your body. Most people benefit from filling their plates with fresh produce, lean proteins, and whole grains, and their glasses with enough water to keep themselves well hydrated. However, it's important not to go overboard and create a plan that's hard to follow or that will just make you feel frustrated and deprived. An eating strategy will be successful and sustainable only if it's custom-made for you and if you enjoy the food you're eating.

THE BENEFITS OF CLEAN EATING

So why would you want to try Clean Eating? People usually start eating cleanly in order to become healthier. Eliminating many of the food additives and groups that are detrimental to your body can result in changes that range from small to lifesaving. The old saying "you are what you eat" is pretty accurate: if you eat junk, your body will eventually fall apart. The flip side of that equation is that eating healthful foods will make your body healthy. Since everyone is unique, the benefits of eating cleanly aren't set in stone. However, people have been doing it long enough that compelling patterns have emerged. Some of the benefits of Clean Eating include:

- Glowing, clear skin
- Lustrous hair
- Improved immunity
- Better sleep
- Loss of body fat
- Increased muscle mass
- Increased energy
- Improved cholesterol and blood sugar levels
- Better mood and improved mental clarity
- Decreased risk of diseases such as cancer, heart disease, diabetes, and stroke
- General feeling of good health

  Bonus benefits include:

- Decreased grocery bills
- Feeling full rather than starved
- Not having to count calories, fat, carbs, or points
- Not having to buy expensive prepackaged foods
- Feeling more confident because you feel better physically

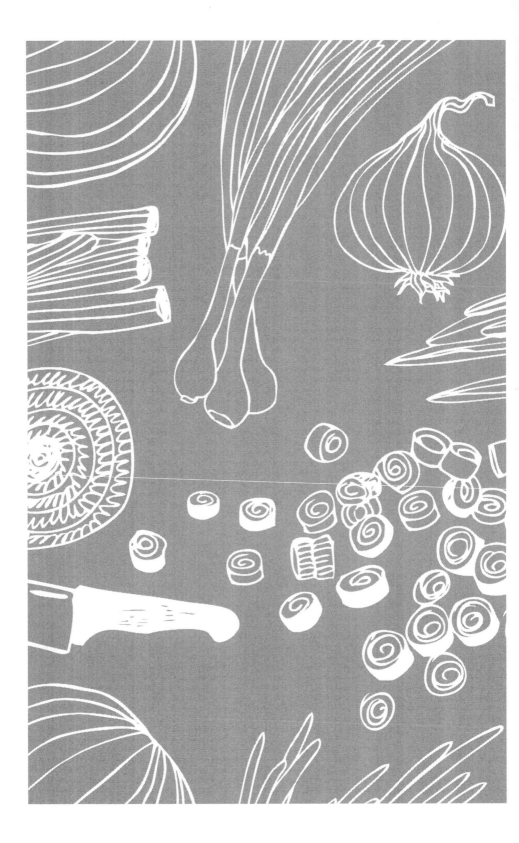

CHAPTER TWO

The Clean Eating Diet

Now that you know what Clean Eating is, you're probably wondering about the nuts and bolts of the plan. There are foods that you eat, foods that you don't, and strategies you can employ to get the best nutritional benefits from your natural food choices. Clean Eating isn't hard to follow once you throw away any preconceptions about carbohydrates, fat, and calories, and instead focus on the fresh, delicious ingredient options. Learning to shop (and eat) cleanly is just a matter of simplifying what you put in your body and making meals that provide you with energy and high-quality fuel. This is mindful eating that takes into account each season's freshest ingredients, powerful food combinations, and super foods to eat at every meal.

FILL YOUR PLATE WITH THE GOOD STUFF

Food is the key to good health. If you choose wholesome, natural foods and follow a balanced meal plan, then you'll have clear skin, shiny hair, and a body at its best, healthiest weight. Clean Eating offers so many food choices that you'll never run out of amazing, diverse dishes for all your meals.

You could be a high achiever who manages to stick to your meal plan 100 percent, but probably not. That's okay—don't obsess over perfection to the point that it makes you miserable. Try to practice your Clean Eating principles 80 percent of the time, and understand that having a small serving of your grandmother's pasta at a family event isn't the end of the world. Just start fresh the next day and don't overindulge when you do make the choice to "cheat."

So what should you put on your plate when following the Clean Eating plan? It's really quite simple at the core. Choose the macronutrients that your body loves best: complex carbohydrates, lean proteins, and good fats. Complex carbs will be the foundation of your diet, to which you'll add protein and good fats. The appendix contains an extensive list of Clean Eating foods, but here are some examples of what you should be eating.

NUTRITION RULES

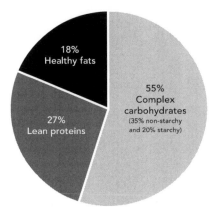

Complex Carbohydrates: Six to Ten Servings per Day

Carbohydrates come in two forms: simple and complex. Most simple carbo-hydrates aren't allowed on the Clean Eating plan, but some fruits (which are simple carbohydrates) are accepted in limited quantities because they're also fantastic sources of fiber and micronutrients such as vitamins and min-erals. Complex carbohydrates like those in the lists that follow are extremely beneficial for your body. They stabilize blood sugar, improve digestion, boost energy, and reduce food cravings (Harvard School of Public Health Nutrition Source 2012).

Non-Starchy Complex Carbohydrates (lower in carbohydrates and calories)

- Apples
- Artichokes
- Asparagus
- Beet greens
- Berries
- Broccoli
- Brussels sprouts
- Cabbage
- Cauliflower
- Celery
- Cucumbers
- Eggplant
- Green beans
- Kale
- Onions
- Spinach
- Swiss chard
- Tomatoes
- Watercress
- Zucchini

Have you ever picked a tomato straight from the vine in your garden, still warm from the sun, and bitten into it like an apple? The taste will simply explode in your mouth with that sweet earthiness that fresh tomatoes are famous for all over the world. Seasonal produce tastes better: it's a fact.

Starchy Complex Carbohydrates

- Bananas
- Beans*
- Brown rice
- Buckwheat
- Bulgur
- Carrots
- Chickpeas*
- Lentils*
- Millet
- Oats
- Potatoes
- Quinoa*
- Radishes
- Split peas*
- Sweet potatoes
- Wheat germ
- Yams

*Can also be used as a source of protein

Lean Protein: Five to Six Servings per Day

The word *protein* is derived from the Greek word for "first," which makes sense because this nutrient is fundamental to the body. Protein is found in all cells of the body and is absolutely crucial for bodily functions. The enzymes in the body that activate chemical processes and many hormones, such as insulin, are proteins. Proteins are made up of about twenty amino acids, nine of which are essential to make a "complete protein" that satisfies all of your body's protein needs. Humans usually get their protein from meats, fish, poultry, and eggs, but it can also be found in other food groups. Some dairy, grains, and vegetables also have substantial amounts of protein. Vegetables often need to be consumed in combination with other foods in order to be a complete protein.

Lean Proteins

- Almond milk
- Beef
- Bison/buffalo
- Cottage cheese, low-fat
- Eggs
- Fish, fresh or low-sodium, water-packed canned
- Kefir (yogurt drink)

- Nut butters
- Nuts (unsalted)
- Pork tenderloin
- Poultry
- Rice milk
- Seeds (hemp, sesame, sunflower, flax, pumpkin)
- Soy milk
- Tempeh
- Tofu
- Yogurt, nonfat

Good Fats (monounsaturated fats and polyunsaturated fats): Two to Three Servings per Day

Many people, especially chronic dieters, are afraid of fat—but, in fact, 18 percent of your daily calories should come in the form of good fats in order for your body to run efficiently. Foods that are good sources of monounsaturated fats can help lower cholesterol and balance blood sugar. This means that eating monounsaturated fats can cut the risk of cardiovascular disease and diabetes. Polyunsaturated fats are mostly vegetable-based and have the same benefits as other healthful fats. Omega-3 fatty acids are polyunsaturated fats that are known for being heart-healthy.

It might be difficult to accept that fat isn't the enemy and that good fats from fish, nuts, olive oil, eggs, some dairy products, and avocados are very healthful for you. You can't live without fat, because it's fuel for your body, it delivers fat-soluble vitamins to your organs, and it provides essential fatty acids. Good fats (polyunsaturated fatty acids and monounsaturated fats) can also help lower cholesterol and reduce the risk of cardiovascular disease. Good fats include:

- Avocados
- Cold-water fish
- Flaxseed
- Hazelnut oil
- Nut butters
- Nuts
- Olive oil
- Pumpkinseed oil
- Safflower oil
- Sunflower seeds

FOODS TO DITCH ON A CLEAN DIET

Clean Eating is about positively choosing good food, not about negatively forbidding or restricting bad food. Obviously, though, there are foods that you'll need to cut out of your diet in order to reap the benefits of a Clean Eating lifestyle. Some will be difficult to give up, especially if they're a habit for you, but don't despair: after eating clean, delicious foods for a while, you won't miss your old diet.

If you dedicate yourself to Clean Eating, you'll have about two thousand opportunities a year to fuel your body with delicious, nutritious foods rather than foods that damage your body. Clean Eating takes the guesswork out of those choices and equips you for a healthier future. Why waste all those chances to get it right?

Conventionally Grown Produce

You should consider cutting out conventionally grown fruits and vegetables, which are contaminated to some degree with chemical fertilizers and pesticides. However, you don't necessarily have to eat organic to eat clean. It might be hard for you to find organic products or they might not be in your budget. If that's the case, make sure you wash your produce well, and choose hormone-, steroid-, and antibiotic-free meats, eggs, and dairy products whenever possible. But you should definitely consider buying certain organic produce—specific foods that are especially contaminated with chemical fertilizers and pesticides when they're grown conventionally (EWG's 2013 Shopper's Guide to Pesticides in Produce 2013). These include:

- Apples
- Bell peppers
- Celery
- Cherry tomatoes
- Collard greens
- Cucumbers
- Grapes
- Hot peppers
- Kale
- Nectarines (imported)
- Peaches
- Potatoes
- Spinach
- Strawberries
- Zucchini

All of these are used in Clean Eating recipes, so you'll need to decide whether or not you want to buy organic.

Processed Foods

Ditch processed foods. This is an essential Clean Eating rule, and following it should be one of the first steps that you take to a healthier life. What counts as processed food? Quite simply, it's anything with unrecognizable ingredients on the label. This means food additives—stuff that's put into food to alter or enhance its flavor, texture, color, shelf life, and even nutritional value. It's disturbing to note that the average North American consumes approximately 150 pounds of food additives a year (Mckee 2008) by eating processed foods.

Processed foods contain:

- Acids (citric, fumaric, lactic, malic, tartaric)
- Antibiotics
- Anticaking agents
- Antifoaming agents
- Artificial flavors
- Artificial sweeteners
- Chemicals
- Dyes
- Emulsifiers
- Flavor enhancers (such as monosodium glutamate)
- Hormones (i.e., rBGH)
- Humectants (keeps processed foods moist and prevents dried foods from drying out too much)
- Preservatives
- Propellants
- Salt
- Stabilizers
- Steroids
- Sugar
- Thickeners
- And many more additives

These ingredients don't belong in a Clean Eating lifestyle. You don't have to cut out every last food item that contains any additives at all, especially when it's otherwise pretty healthful, like whole-grain tortillas. But do your very best.

Refined Sugar

Refined sugar is nothing but empty calories, which not only packs on the pounds but also damages your health. Bottom line: you should never eat refined sugar again. The standard American diet is absolutely overloaded with sugar, not just in desserts and candy but also in many items that you might assume are sugar-free, such as store-bought spaghetti sauce, deli meats, and canned soup. Sugar consumption substantially increases the risk of many deadly diseases, such as diabetes, heart disease, high blood pressure, and high triglyceride levels, not to mention obesity (Jacob 2013).

Refined Grains

All grain products aren't created equal, even though they start out that way in the fields. White flour is the world's most common refined grain and is found absolutely everywhere, such as in cereal, breads, cakes, pizza, sauces, soups, cookies, and muffins. When nutritious whole wheat is processed, it turns into a starchy powder that can cause numerous health problems, including elevated blood sugar, sugar cravings, sluggish metabolism, inflammation, and allergic reactions to gluten (see the glossary) (Women Fitness 2011). The Clean Eating plan replaces this damaging food with whole grains that still have all the edible parts of the entire grain kernel, including the bran, the germ, and the endosperm.

Trans Fats and Saturated Fats

These fats are often found in processed foods because manufacturers use them to create a desirable characteristic known as "mouth feel," a pleasant texture in the mouth. Fats also can add flavor.

Trans fats are completely artificial—they're not found in nature—and should never pass your lips. They contribute to many dangerous health conditions such as coronary heart disease and obesity.

Saturated fats are more of a gray area because you can occasionally consume them in very small quantities (Teicholz 2007). Saturated fats usually come from animal sources, such as meat and milk, and are solid at room temperature—think butter and lard. Eating too much saturated fat can increase your risk of several chronic diseases, such as breast and colon cancer, and contribute to obesity (Collins 2012).

Specific Foods to Cut from Your Diet

Eliminate refined sugar, refined grain, and bad fats from your diet by permanently crossing foods like these off your shopping list:

- Beverages: energy drinks; fruit cocktails, drinks, and bottled juices (eat fresh fruit instead); sodas; sweetened or creamy coffee drinks
- Condiments: full-fat mayonnaise; most store-bought sauces, dressings, and marinades
- Dairy products: butter; hard cheeses
- Fried foods, including French fries
- Frozen foods: breakfasts, dinners, pizza, snacks
- Hydrogenated oils
- Meats: bacon; fatty cuts of beef; ground beef; ham; hamburgers; hot dogs; most lamb; processed deli meats; sausages
- Palm oil
- Pastries: cakes; cookies; donuts; pies; snack cakes
- Pizza

- Refined grains: white breads; pasta; and rice
- Salty snacks: chips; crackers
- Stick margarine
- Sugary breakfast cereals
- Sweets: candy, ice cream, marshmallow spread, milk chocolate

FOOD PAIRING: BEYOND PEAS AND CARROTS

One of most important principles of Clean Eating is to combine lean proteins and complex carbohydrates in every meal. This food formula helps stabilize blood sugar, eliminating the nasty symptoms of fluctuating levels of sugar-regulating insulin, such as dizziness, sweat, food cravings, and energy crashes (Worden 2011). Food pairing also leaves you feeling full longer between meals and provides fuel for exercising and everyday activities.

You can also combine Clean Eating foods to enhance the absorption rate of the nutrients. These combinations involve specific foods, but more often they pair complementary nutrients. Experiment with different foods and you might hit upon a new favorite taste.

Ten Perfect Clean Eating Pairings

1. **Tomatoes + avocados:** This could be the base of a delicious salad or tempting guacamole. The good fat in the avocado makes your body absorb seven times more of the lycopene (an antioxidant; see the glossary) in the tomatoes. Plus, the fat-soluble vitamins in tomatoes need a source of good fat—the avocado—to be absorbed by your body.
2. **Dark green vegetables + extra-virgin olive oil:** The olive oil helps release the antioxidant lutein that's found in the vegetables (Roodenburg et al. 2000).
3. **Cruciferous vegetables + grilled proteins:** There's a great deal of concern about carcinogens that are formed during high-heat cooking such as grilling. Cauliflower, Brussels sprouts, kale, and broccoli contain compounds that can help your body purge the carcinogens in grilled foods (National Cancer Institute 2012).
4. **Spinach + citrus fruit:** If you have anemia or low blood iron, this combination might be the solution for you. Adding orange wedges to your fresh spinach salad will help your body absorb the iron in the greens more

readily (Roodenburg et al. 2000). You can also dress the salad or cooked greens with a squeeze of fresh lemon or lime juice.

5. **Greek yogurt + whole grains or bananas:** Imagine eating a dish that provides your body with healthful digestive bacteria (probiotics) and the food that those bacteria thrive on (prebiotics). In this case, the prebiotics in the grains or bananas combine with the probiotics in the yogurt to help your digestive system stay healthy and run smoothly.

6. **Tomatoes and broccoli + extra-virgin olive oil:** Tomatoes and broccoli are wonderful sources of beta-carotene, which can help your body fight off colds if it's absorbed well. This is where the olive oil comes into the equation: monounsaturated fat such as olive oil can increase the absorption of beta-carotene by 500 percent.

7. **Whole-grain pasta + roasted bell peppers:** Most people don't realize that whole-grain pasta is a great source of iron, but it isn't easily absorbed by your body. However, the vitamin C in roasted bell peppers helps convert the iron into a form that your body can easily access (Worden 2011). It's a real energy boost, which makes pasta-plus-peppers a great pre-workout meal.

8. **Wild salmon + kale:** Have you ever wondered why dairy producers enrich milk with vitamin D? It's because your body needs vitamin D to absorb calcium. In this pairing, the vitamin D in the wild salmon helps your body absorb the calcium in the kale.

9. **Mushrooms + salmon:** Mushrooms are a good source of niacin (vitamin B_3), which can help enhance the anti-inflammatory and triglyceride-lowering effects of the fish oil in salmon. This is a great recipe for lowering bad cholesterol and raising good cholesterol.

10. **Whole grains + garlic:** This combination is the perfect base for an absolutely delicious casserole, but it can also boost your immune system. Garlic is a source of sulfur, which can substantially improve the absorption of the zinc in whole grains.

SEASONAL EATING: APPLES IN FALL, CITRUS IN WINTER

One of the best strategies when eating cleanly is to eat seasonally. When you buy foods that are in season, you're generally buying items that are grown locally and picked shortly before they're sold. Depending on where you live, you might not be able to find all of your seasonal produce locally, but most parts of the country do have at least some local crops available at supermarkets, farm stands, farmers' markets, and community-supported agriculture (CSA) memberships. You might also consider growing some vegetables and fruit yourself, if you can, for the ultimate in local eating. To add seasonal items to your Clean Eating plan, go online and look up sources of seasonal produce in your area. Buying food seasonally and locally has become so popular that it's now easy to find information.

Unless you live in an area with a mild climate that supports farming year-round, you won't have access to a wide variety of local crops in every season. If that's the case, look for produce that's grown as close to you as possible—for instance, in California rather than Chile. There are many reasons to eat food that's in season:

- **Cost:** Locally grown and picked foods are usually less expensive than those shipped from a distance, because it costs less to get them to market. For the most part, foods grown outdoors rather than in greenhouses also cost less to produce, and that savings is passed on to the consumer.
- **Taste:** Have you ever inhaled the heady fragrance of a ripe, blushing peach in a farmers' market, then bitten into its sweet, juicy flesh right after buying it? Seasonal produce tastes better—it's a fact. When a tomato is produced in a hothouse thousands of miles away, it's picked almost green so it doesn't bruise as easily in the trucks. Then it's chemically treated to give it the desirable red color, which means it really isn't ripe. More likely, it will feel mealy and lack flavor. The tomato might not even be very red. Chilling, transporting, and sitting in warehouses leaches the flavor and nutrition right out of the fruit and vegetables sold out of season or far from where they're grown. By contrast, fresh, seasonal, local produce still bursts with full flavor, juiciness, and nutritional value.
- **Variety:** Depending on where you live and what season it is, you might be amazed at the large selection of seasonal produce available. Each season offers a long list of products that you can find in supermarkets and farmers' markets. There's even seasonal produce in the winter, when leeks, dark leafy greens, radishes, and citrus fruits abound.
- **Nutrition:** You might be appalled to learn what happens to most non-seasonal produce on its journey to market. That healthy bright bag of spinach you just bought might not contain all its nutrients by the time

you put it on your plate, and it might contain stuff that you really don't want to eat. Some of the indignities it may have suffered include irradiation (to kill bugs) and treatment with preservatives (such as wax), which are meant to protect the produce during long trips.

FIFTY SUPER FOODS

The best Clean Eating foods are "super foods" packed full of healthful vitamins, minerals, antioxidants, essential fatty acids, and phytonutrients (see the glossary). Many Clean Eating recipes feature super foods in tasty combinations, maximizing their wide variety of health benefits. Include super foods in your Clean Eating meal plans every day to reap their benefits. Super foods can:

- Help stabilize blood sugar
- Reduce the risk of cardiovascular disease by reducing bad cholesterol, increasing good cholesterol, and lowering blood pressure
- Reduce or prevent inflammation
- Reduce the risk of certain cancers
- Strengthen immunity
- Increase metabolism and support weight loss
- Purge toxins from your body
- Promote good digestive health

Here's a list of fifty super foods, most of which you can easily find in your supermarket or at your farmers' market, no matter where you live. This isn't a comprehensive list by any means, but rather a compilation of some especially good examples. These super foods are constantly changing, so you might find completely different lists online and in health-related books. All the foods listed will be nutritious and beneficial to the body. Try to consume them fresh and in season whenever possible.

- Alliums (garlic, onion, shallot, scallion, leeks, chives)
- Apples
- Artichokes
- Asparagus
- Avocados
- Bananas
- Beans
- Beets
- Berries (strawberries, blueberries, goji, blackberries, cranberries, acai)
- Broccoli
- Brown rice

- Brussels sprouts
- Cabbage
- Carrots
- Cauliflower
- Cherries
- Dark chocolate
- Dark leafy greens (kale, spinach, beet greens, collard greens, Swiss chard)
- Eggs
- Fish
- Grapes
- Greek yogurt, low-fat, nonfat
- Green tea
- Herbs
- Hot peppers
- Kiwis
- Kukicha twig tea
- Lemons
- Mangoes
- Melons (watermelon, cantaloupe, honeydew)
- Mushrooms
- Nuts
- Oats
- Olive oil
- Oranges
- Papayas
- Peaches
- Pineapples
- Pumpkins
- Pomegranates
- Quinoa
- Rhubarb
- Salmon
- Seeds (pumpkin, sesame, sunflower, chai, hemp, flax)
- Spirulina
- Squash
- Sweet potatoes
- Tomatoes
- Tuna
- Wheat germ

CHAPTER THREE

Getting Started with Clean Eating

There are some basic principles for the Clean Eating plan, but it's definitely not a rigid diet that forbids variations. The plan accommodates health, logistical, and everyday situations that might crop up. Clean Eating is meant to be a lifestyle that you'll be delighted to follow for the rest of your life, one that can be tailored to fit your needs and routine. Nothing derails a change in eating patterns faster than inconvenience, complexity, or hard-to-find ingredients. Follow the essential rules as much as possible, but cut yourself some slack when you're not perfect. Here are the fundamentals.

CLEAN EATING DOS AND DON'TS

- **Do eat lots of fresh fruits and vegetables:** Clean Eating is all about whole foods like fresh produce. Top your cereal with fresh berries or a banana, eat salads that combine many colors and textures, and toss steamed vegetables with chunks of lean skinless, boneless chicken or whole-grain pasta for a satisfying dinner. Fruits and vegetables are a wonderful addition to any meal or snack.
- **Do eat five to six small meals a day instead of three large meals:** Spreading your meals out evenly from when you get up to when you go to bed prevents blood sugar spikes and reduces cravings. Starving yourself or eating three big meals a day can create real blood sugar issues, so consistency is the key to success. Fueling your body constantly with nutrient-rich foods revs up your metabolism to give you constant energy all day. Try to eat every two to three hours, and never skip a meal. Anyone who has experienced the dreaded midafternoon energy slump will tell you that low blood sugar can wreak havoc on your body. When you hit that wall with no healthful food in sight, a sugary, fattening snack often

seems to be the only solution. Refined sugar might help initially, but your blood glucose high will eventually crash—even more dramatically—later in the day. The best solution is to keep your body from reaching metabolic extremes. Always eat breakfast to kick-start your metabolism and start the day off right. Then eat several smaller, nutritious meals every few hours. At first, even though you're not eating the refined carbs and saturated fats that you're used to, you might actually find that you feel too full. But don't skip any meals! Doing so will eventually lead to weight gain because it slows down your metabolism.

- **Do drink lots of water:** Most people know that the human body is about 66 percent water and that it can't go very long without water. This vital liquid does a great deal of good in your body. It flushes toxins, helps with the absorption of nutrients, assists with regulating body temperature, and supports lustrous hair and glowing skin. "Drink lots of water" has been a health mantra for decades. When it comes to Clean Eating, staying hydrated throughout the day, especially when exercising, is key. When you're thirsty, you're dehydrated. Properly hydrated muscles perform better and you'll be less apt to feel sore the day after you work out.

- **Do carry clean food with you:** You should never get caught without a stash of clean food, both when you're out and when you're home. If you do, you might skip a meal or eat something that isn't good for you. Keep lots of clean food in your fridge, prepared ahead of time, and invest in a cooler that you can pack with leftovers, fruit, nuts, and bottles of water. Soon this will become a routine and you'll breeze through your day with no food mistakes.

- **Do start your day with fresh lemon juice squeezed into a cup of hot water:** Many Asian cultures advocate beginning the day with water and lemon to detoxify the liver (Gucciardi 2012). Your liver filters toxins from your blood, so maintaining this hard-working organ is a step in the right direction. Drinking lemon and hot water first thing in the morning can also hydrate you after sleeping and cut the amount of coffee you drink.

- **Do add exercise to your routine:** Cardio (aerobic) exercise and weight training are definitely important components of Clean Eating, because exercise is part of creating a healthier body. Get your heart pumping and oxygen flowing with cardio exercise that puts your body in motion, such as brisk walking, dancing, competitive and individual sports, swimming, and even climbing the stairs instead of taking the elevator. Weight training builds muscle, which revs up your metabolism, increases stamina, and helps you develop an attractive, toned physique. Getting in shape will also boost your confidence.

- **Do eat both complex carbohydrates and protein at every meal:** This Clean Eating essential is set in stone because pairing your foods this way can prevent fluctuations in your insulin levels, reduce food cravings, help with weight-loss goals, promote fat burning, and increase energy (Venuto 2009). With so many foods to choose from in each nutritional category, it's very easy to come up with tasty pairings. Proteins can include skinless, boneless chicken; fish; lean meats; nut butters; and legumes. Complex carbohydrates are fresh vegetables and fruits and whole grains.

- **Don't skimp on sleep:** There never seem to be enough hours in the day to get everything done, and sometimes sleep isn't a priority. But sleep is vital to losing weight and maintaining a healthy body. When you sleep, your body produces human growth hormone, which stimulates your metabolism (Hensrud 2012). Sleep deprivation robs you of energy to exercise or even to engage in ordinary daily activities. And if you're exhausted, it's more likely you'll reach for easy but temporary energy fixes like sugary foods and caffeinated beverages. That's bad for your health and bad for your weight.

- **Don't ever skip meals:** Anyone who has dieted to lose weight has tried skipping meals to cut calories. This doesn't work, and it's one of the reasons diets often fail (Tomiyama et al. 2010). When you skip meals, your blood sugar fluctuates wildly, which leads to cravings, lack of energy, and overeating.

- **Don't forget that food is nutritional medicine:** Eating is definitely a pleasure, but never lose sight of the fact that food is meant to support and fuel your body efficiently. What you put in your mouth can either benefit you or create health issues. Eating clean, nutrient-packed foods is crucial for optimal health and will help establish a strong foundation for wellness throughout your life.

- **Don't start your week without a Clean Eating meal plan:** Clean Eating is all about mindful eating and carefully choosing what foods to put in your body. Without a plan it's difficult to shop wisely, prepare clean meals, and pack your cooler for when you're out of the house. The old saying "failing to plan means planning to fail" holds true in the Clean Eating lifestyle.

- **Don't eat high-sodium foods:** Eating less sodium can actually cut your risk of cardiovascular disease by about 25 to 30 percent, because sodium intake is linked to high blood pressure (PsychEducation 2003). Most processed foods are a huge source of sodium, so they're no-no's on the Clean Eating plan. In addition, it's important to use herbs and spices rather than salt to boost the flavor when preparing your meals. Adding salt to your food is often a habit more than a flavor preference, so try cooking without it—you might be surprised at how delicious food tastes on its own.
- **Don't leave the house unprepared:** Always bring along a cooler of clean foods and healthful meals. And always carry plenty of water wherever you go. You never know if you might get stuck in traffic or if that appointment will take longer than expected. It's a good idea to pack your containers the night before—dinner leftovers make a tasty lunch—so that you can fly out the door prepared for a hectic day.

THE IMPORTANCE OF EXERCISE

Choosing clean, wholesome foods is only one component of Clean Eating; you also should include exercise in your daily routine. Experts recommend that you do a minimum of thirty minutes of aerobic exercise three days a week, and work your way up to as much as sixty minutes five to six times per week. It's especially important to train with weights at least three times a week.

There are good reasons why Clean Eating has been an element of body-building culture for decades. When you move, your body undergoes a process called lipolysis, which frees fat from your fat cells (Goto et al. 2007). Exercise also releases testosterone, which breaks down fat for hours after your workout ends. Cardio exercise is important, but weight training is particularly beneficial, especially if you're trying to lose weight. Lifting weights can actually sculpt your body, and working your big muscle groups fires up your metabolism as all those muscle fibers contract hundreds of times. But be careful not to overtrain, which can cause injuries and destroy all your forward progress. Overtraining can cause fatigue, depression, and underperformance of your exercises. Slowly work up to intense, focused sessions for less than an hour a day and rest in between. The way you feel and look comes only 10 percent from exercise, while genetics counts for another 10 percent, and nutrition accounts for the remaining 80 percent (Reno 2006).

The benefits of regular exercise include:

- Weight loss or decreased body fat
- A more efficient metabolism—muscle burns more energy at rest
- Fewer hunger pangs and food cravings; exercise is a natural appetite suppressant
- A toned, tighter body
- Increased energy
- A stronger immune system and a reduced chance of getting chronic illnesses
- Improved cardiovascular functioning
- Better lung capacity
- Deep, satisfying sleep
- Increased sex drive
- Healthy skin

Remember, it's important to consult with your health care provider before starting any exercise program.

TEN STEPS TO GET STARTED

1. Make a commitment to yourself and find support.

Clean Eating is a lifestyle choice that requires a commitment to a healthier you. Your goals can be reached only if you commit to yourself. It can be very difficult to put yourself first and understand that doing so isn't selfish. Your commitment to Clean Eating will actually take your relationships with your family, friends, and coworkers to a higher level. It's also important to tell people your plans and to seek support with your goals. This is a wonderful way to stay on track . . . and you never know who might want to join you!

2. Write down your goals and keep a journal.

At the beginning of your Clean Eating journey it's very important to document what you want to achieve, such as losing twenty pounds, lowering your cholesterol by a certain number of points, or taking your body mass index (BMI) down to a particular number. Be as specific as possible and set realistic milestones so that you have a clear focus and can create a game plan around those goals. Write down what you eat every day, along with your exercise schedule and anything else that gives you insight into your eating habits. For example, you might write down that you get really hungry or have flagging energy in the afternoon. This means you should eat something a little more substantial as a snack.

3. Start with a clean slate.

When you make the decision to eat cleanly, you need to clean all of the bad food out of your fridge, cupboards, pantry, car, and "secret places." This might seem like a waste of money, but you need to remove all temptations. You can give the food to relatives or even donate it to a food bank if you don't want to fill up garbage bags. Remember to toss condiments, cereals, and hidden stashes of old Halloween candy.

4. Have a plan when you shop for food.

Never go shopping without a meal plan and shopping list in hand, and stick to the list even if other items are on sale. And don't go to the supermarket hungry! Eat something before hitting the supermarket: research has shown that hungry shoppers buy more food as well as more junk convenience foods. But the most important shopping tip is to read the label of every product you want to buy to find any ingredients that aren't on the Clean Eating list.

5. Avoid foods with ingredients you don't recognize.

If you've ever spent time studying labels on food products, you know that many of the ingredients of popular foods sound like the makings of a chemistry experiment. This isn't too far from the truth. These unrecognizable ingredients are used as preservatives, to add color, to stop products from clumping, and for many other reasons. A good Clean Eating strategy is to either buy whole, single ingredients or to look for products that have few ingredients. Foods that contain lots of empty calories make up the bulk of the standard American diet (SAD), and many people aren't aware of how much bad food they consume. Even foods that are advertised as healthful, such as frozen diet dinners and "light" foods, are packed with ingredients that can harm your health. A good Clean Eating rule of thumb is to purchase only fresh foods or those with the shortest list of ingredients—"real" ingredients, that is—on their labels. If you can't spell or pronounce something, there's a good chance that you shouldn't eat it, either.

6. Accept that you'll probably be eating more food rather than less.

Don't panic when you look at the amount of food you'll be carrying around and enjoying when eating cleanly. Eating more to lose weight might seem like a strange concept, but it makes sense when you consider how unstable blood sugar and binge eating affect your body. It's also infinitely better to fill up on healthful whole foods rather than indulge in junk food. So follow your meal plans without skipping meals or counting calories, and trust your body to use all those nutrients effectively.

7. Remember that your body is unique.

On the Clean Eating plan, strive to be the best you rather than trying to look like anyone else. Every single person in the world has different needs when it comes to nutrition, exercise, and health. This is a lifestyle choice, not a diet, and for the best results you need to tailor it to your situation and body. If you have a health condition such as diabetes, you'll need to take that into account when planning your meals, even though Clean Eating is very beneficial for people with diabetes.

8. Drink lots of water.

Water is often not the first choice for people when they're thirsty. But on the Clean Eating plan it's important to drink as much water as you can. This is probably one of the simpler steps to take, and if you really don't like water, you can jazz it up with a fresh squeeze of lemon, lime, or orange juice. If you haven't been a big water drinker, you might be pleasantly surprised to find that your headaches, fatigue, and dull skin disappear when you start hydrating more. Hydrating your body properly will make you feel better immediately.

9. Stop eating sugar, saturated fats, refined foods, and junk foods.

Cutting out all the foods that are bad for you will create monumental positive changes in your body almost immediately. On the Clean Eating plan, you should completely avoid sugar because it can sabotage your health goals. Clean Eating isn't really about forbidden foods; it's about foods that don't contain refined sugar in their natural states, even sweet fruit. Sugar causes catastrophic effects in your body, such as soaring blood sugar, deep energy and mental crashes, and intense food cravings. Too much sugar in your diet can cause high blood pressure, diabetes, and obesity (Hyman 2012). Read your labels closely to look for hidden sugar, such as in spaghetti sauce or bread, and satisfy your sweet tooth with a natural treat like pineapple raisins. When you avoid sugar, refined foods, and junk foods, you might lose weight, experience fewer mood swings, and have sharper mental focus. However, in some cases, this type of food purge results in withdrawal symptoms such as headaches or fatigue, especially if sugar is a major component of your diet. Don't give up if this occurs: the backlash is temporary, and it means you're on the right track. Just keep your goals at the forefront of your mind and stick with it.

10. Eat more fresh produce, lean protein, and whole grains.

Instead of packaged convenience items, fill your grocery cart with a plethora of fresh, vibrant produce in as many colors as possible. Add lean protein sources (the most healthful are organic and free-range, but if you can't find or afford those, at least try to find hormone-, steroid-, and antibiotic-free protein), and round out your list with whole-grain products. Shoot for a cart that contains very few boxes, jars, or cans. Since switching to whole, nutritious foods is what Clean Eating is all about, this is the most important step to take in order to get started on your new lifestyle. "Whole" doesn't refer to an entire apple or carrot (although these are whole foods!), but rather to foods that are as close to their natural state as possible. Such foods are whole because nothing has been removed from them through processing or refining. When they're refined, grains and other carbohydrates are stripped of vitamins, minerals, and fiber; they still contain calories, but they've lost their nutrients. Beyond whole wheat, you can buy all kinds of whole grains, from barley and oats to quinoa and wild rice. Look for the word "whole" before the ingredients on products such as bread, flour, breakfast cereal, and tortillas. These healthful grains reduce the risk of heart disease and help keep your blood sugar stable (Worden 2011). Think of natural, whole foods this way: a bowl of blueberries and steel-cut oatmeal makes a much more healthful breakfast than an oatmeal-blueberry muffin (which is most likely filled with sugar and other harmful ingredients). Whenever possible, prepare and cook your own whole foods rather than eating processed foods.

CHAPTER FOUR

14-Day Clean Eating Meal Plan

This simple but comprehensive fourteen-day meal plan shows you how to put the Clean Eating guidelines into practice. Keep in mind that it's an example of what two weeks of Clean Eating could look like, but it isn't written in stone. Every meal outlined here is unique and complete, but you could choose instead to make your lunch out of the leftovers from last night's dinner. (It's actually a good idea to do so, because it will save time when you're packing your Clean Eating cooler for work or school.) Another way to tweak the plan is to swap out dessert for a very light snack a couple of hours after dinner. It's up to you!

Most, if not all, of the ingredients in this meal plan should be quite familiar and easy to find at your supermarket. You won't have to search the Internet to find an Asian foods website or Latin American culinary glossary. Keep in mind that you can substitute a clean ingredient or recipe that you like better than one that's in the meal plan. For example, if you really like quinoa or bulgur, you can have that instead of rice where specified in the meal plan. You can even experiment—for instance, with other interesting grains and different flour substitutes—to add new dimension to your dishes. This approach will make it easier and more fun to follow the Clean Eating lifestyle.

The two weekly shopping lists include all the ingredients that you'll need for each week. Check your pantry and fridge to see what you already have, and cross those items off your list so you don't buy more than you need. Ingredients that frequently fall into this category include vanilla extract, hot sauce, mustard, flour, rice, dried beans, herbs, spices, salt, and pepper, which are not usually used up in one recipe.

Note: Dishes marked with a asterisk (*) are provided in the recipe section.

DAY 1

Breakfast

2 poached eggs on a whole-grain bagel

2 tablespoons chopped tomato

1 orange

Midmorning snack

2 carrots

1 tablespoon nut butter

Lunch

*Lemon Brown Rice Salad

Midafternoon snack

1 apple

10 unsalted almonds

Dinner

6 ounces broiled or grilled skinless, boneless chicken breast

1 baked potato

2 tablespoons cottage cheese

1 cup steamed green beans

Dessert

*Smooth Lime Pudding

DAY 2

Breakfast

1 cup *Clean Eating Granola

Midmorning snack

¾ cup nonfat plain Greek yogurt

¼ cup sunflower seeds

Lunch

*Mushroom Beet Green Salad

Midafternoon snack

1 whole-grain tortilla

1 tablespoon nut butter

½ cup grapes

Dinner

5 ounces grilled sirloin steak

¾ cup cooked quinoa

12 grilled asparagus spears

Dessert

1 cup unsweetened applesauce

1 tablespoon chopped pecans

DAY 3

Breakfast

2 scrambled eggs

1 piece whole-wheat toast

1 tomato, sliced

1 banana

Midmorning snack

2 *Oatmeal Raisin Cookies

Lunch

Chicken Romaine Salad

- 6 ounces broiled or grilled skinless, boneless chicken breast, sliced
- 2 cups chopped spinach
- ½ cup halved cherry tomatoes
- ½ cup sliced cucumber
- ¼ avocado, peeled, pitted, and sliced
- 1 teaspoon apple cider vinegar

Midafternoon snack

2 kiwis

10 pecan halves

Dinner

*Baked Halibut Vegetable Casserole

Dessert

*Peach Cobbler

DAY 4

Breakfast

*Rhubarb Bread Pudding for the Slow Cooker

Midmorning snack

2 large carrots

1 tablespoon almond butter

Lunch

Greek Salad

- ½ cup drained chickpeas
- ½ English cucumber, diced
- 1 tomato, diced
- ¼ cup diced red onion
- 2 tablespoons crumbled low-sodium feta

Midafternoon snack

*Mango Pineapple Ice Pops

Dinner

4 ounces halibut, broiled

Mixed Stir-Fried Vegetables

- 1 teaspoon sesame oil
- ½ cup broccoli florets
- ½ cup cauliflower florets
- ½ cup sliced carrot
- 6 mushrooms, sliced
- ½ red bell pepper, sliced

Dessert

1 cup sliced fresh strawberries

¼ cup sunflower seeds

DAY 5

Breakfast

Quinoa, Almond and Berries

- 1 cup cooked quinoa
- 2 tablespoons skim milk
- 2 tablespoons chopped almonds
- 1 tablespoon dried cranberries

1 peach

Midmorning snack

*Green Energy Smoothie

Lunch

Tuna Wrap

- 1 whole-wheat wrapper (such as a whole-grain tortilla)
- 4 ounces drained low-sodium, water-packed canned tuna

- ½ cup shredded lettuce
- 2 tomato slices

Midafternoon snack

½ cup low-fat plain Greek yogurt

½ cup blueberries

Dinner

Baked Chicken with Peach Salsa

- 4 ounces baked skinless, boneless chicken breast
- Peach Salsa
  - 1 peach, diced
  - ¼ red bell pepper, diced
  - ¼ cup diced cucumber
  - ½ scallion, sliced

½ cup cooked brown rice

1 cup blanched green beans

Dessert

2 (1-ounce) squares dark chocolate

½ cup raspberries

DAY 6

Breakfast

Egg White Scramble

- 3 scrambled egg whites
- ¼ cup diced red bell pepper
- ¼ cup diced onion
- ¼ cup diced zucchini

½ whole-grain bagel

Midmorning snack

*Clean Berry Parfait

Lunch

*Chicken Pecan Salad

Midafternoon snack

1 cup cubed cantaloupe

1 ounce low-fat cheese

Dinner

4 ounces broiled or grilled pork tenderloin

1 cup steamed new potatoes

1 cup steamed cauliflower florets

1 teaspoon chopped almonds

Dessert

Simple Banana Rice Pudding

- ½ cup brown rice, cooked in ½ cup almond milk and ½ cup water
- ½ banana, sliced
- 1 teaspoon maple syrup

DAY 7

Breakfast

1 cup oatmeal

- 1 banana
- 1 tablespoon chopped almonds

1 hardboiled egg

Midmorning snack

*Almond Quinoa Squares

Lunch

Chicken Bagel Sandwich

- 2 ounces baked or broiled skinless, boneless chicken breast
- ½ toasted whole-grain bagel
- ½ teaspoon Dijon mustard
- 1 slice tomato
- 4 slices cucumber

1 peach

Midafternoon snack

1 banana

10 almonds

Dinner

*Sea Scallops with Coconut Curry Sauce

½ cup cooked brown rice

1 cup sliced zucchini, sautéed in ½ teaspoon extra-virgin olive oil

Dessert

Grilled peach halves

½ cup low-fat plain Greek yogurt

DAY 8

Breakfast

*Spanakopita Frittata

Midmorning snack

1 apple

1 tablespoon almond butter

Lunch

*Sunny Carrot Squash Soup

Midafternoon snack

1 cup cubed watermelon

1 ounce low-sodium feta

Dinner

Chicken Penne

- 1 cup cooked whole-wheat penne
- 4 ounces skinless, boneless chicken breast, sliced and sautéed in ½ tea-spoon extra-virgin olive oil
- ½ red bell pepper, sliced thinly
- ½ green bell pepper, sliced thinly
- 1 tomato, diced

Dessert

Strawberry Pudding

- 1 cup strawberries, pureed
- ¼ cup coconut milk
- ½ avocado, peeled, pitted, and sliced

DAY 9

Breakfast

Peanut Butter Banana Wrap

- 1 whole-grain tortilla
- 1 tablespoon natural peanut butter
- ½ banana, sliced

½ grapefruit

Midmorning snack

⅓ cup low-fat cottage cheese

1 slice watermelon

1 tablespoon sunflower seeds

Lunch

Arugula Salad

- 2 hard-boiled eggs, sliced
- 1 cup arugula
- ½ cup cherry tomatoes
- ½ green pepper, sliced
- ½ cup grated carrot
- Freshly squeezed juice of ½ lemon

Midafternoon snack

1 cup broccoli florets

½ avocado, peeled, pitted, and sliced

Dinner

*Roast Pork Loin with Fennel

1 baked sweet potato

Small green salad

- 1 cup mixed greens
- ½ small tomato
- 2 slices red onion
- 4 slices cucumber

Dessert

*Chocolate Pots Crème

DAY 10

Breakfast

1 cup low-fat plain Greek yogurt

- ¼ cup rolled oats
- ½ cup sliced strawberries

½ toasted whole-wheat English muffin

Midmorning snack

1 peach

¼ cup sunflower seeds

Lunch

Tuna Spinach Salad

- 4 ounces low-sodium, water-packed canned tuna
- ½ cup chickpeas
- 2 cups baby spinach
- ½ grapefruit, peeled and cut into segments
- ½ cup halved cherry tomatoes

Midafternoon snack

2 celery stalks

1 tablespoon nut butter

Dinner

6 ounces grilled sirloin steak

1 cup whole-wheat couscous

1 cup blanched green beans sprinkled with nutmeg

Dessert

*Cherry Granita

DAY 11

Breakfast

Brown Rice Hot Cereal

- 1 cup cooked brown rice
- ½ cup almond milk
- Drizzle of honey
- 1 cup chopped pear

Midmorning snack

*Creamy Fruit Dip

Lunch

Chicken Waldorf Salad

- 4 ounces baked or broiled skinless, boneless chicken breast
- 3 celery stalks, sliced
- 1 apple, cored and chopped
- ½ cup halved red grapes
- 10 chopped pecans
- 2 tablespoons nonfat plain Greek yogurt

Midafternoon snack

½ baked sweet potato

10 pecans

Dinner

*Herb-Crusted Pork Chops

2 cups steamed Brussels sprouts

½ cup cooked quinoa

Dessert

½ baked sweet potato, mashed

- Drizzle of maple syrup
- 1 tablespoon chopped pecans

DAY 12

Breakfast
*Simple Egg Wraps

Midmorning snack
1 apple
1 tablespoon almond butter

Lunch
Steak Wraps
- 4 ounces broiled or grilled flank steak
- 1 whole-wheat tortilla
- 1 cup shredded spinach
- 1 tomato, chopped
- 2 tablespoons chopped red onion
- 2 tablespoons crumbled low-sodium feta

1 bunch grapes

Midafternoon snack
1 cup cubed honeydew melon
10 almonds

Dinner
5 ounces broiled or baked tilapia
- Squeeze of fresh lemon

½ cup cooked brown rice
1 cup lightly blanched green beans

Dessert
*Banana Coconut Soft-Serve Ice Cream

DAY 13

Breakfast
1 cup oatmeal
- Drizzle of maple syrup
- 1 cup sliced strawberries
- 1 tablespoon chopped pecans

Midmorning snack
1 banana
2 tablespoons roasted sunflower seeds

Lunch

*Creamy Broccoli Soup

Midafternoon snack

½ whole-wheat English muffin

1 tablespoon nut butter

1 apple

Dinner

Baked Pecan-Crusted Pork Chop

- 5-ounce baked pork chop
- 1 tablespoon crushed pecans

Coleslaw

- 1 cup shredded cabbage
- ½ cup shredded carrot
- ¼ cup thinly sliced red onion
- 1 tablespoon low-fat plain Greek yogurt
- Splash of apple cider vinegar

Dessert

*Baked Apples

DAY 14

Breakfast

Blueberry Smoothie

- 1 cup blueberries
- ½ cup almond milk
- 1 banana
- Handful baby spinach leaves
- 2 ice cubes

Midmorning snack

*Cantaloupe Ice Cream

Lunch

Broccoli-Stuffed Baked Potato

- 1 baked potato, flesh mixed with:
    - ½ cup blanched broccoli florets
    - ¼ cup nonfat cottage cheese
    - ¼ cup diced, baked skinless, boneless chicken breast

Midafternoon snack

3 celery stalks

2 tablespoons nut butter

Dinner

*Curried Chicken Couscous

Dessert

Stuffed Honeydew Melon

- ½ honeydew, seeded
- ½ cup rolled oats
- 3 pecans, chopped
- 2 tablespoons nonfat cottage cheese
- Sprinkle of cinnamon

WEEK 1 SHOPPING LIST

Proteins and Dairy

- 1 carton almond milk
- 5 (6-ounce) skinless, boneless chicken breasts
- 1 can sodium-free chickpeas
- 1 carton coconut milk
- 1 container nonfat cottage cheese
- 1 dozen eggs
- 1 container low-sodium feta
- 5 (6-ounce) halibut fillets
- 1 quart nonfat milk
- 8-ounce pork tenderloin, trimmed of visible fat
- 1 pound cleaned sea scallops
- 1 (5-ounce) sirloin steak
- 1 can low-sodium, water-packed tuna
- 3 (16-ounce) containers nonfat or low-fat plain Greek yogurt

Veggies and Fruit

- 1 apple
- 1 bag arugula

- 12 asparagus spears
- 3 avocados
- 4 bananas
- 1 bunch fresh basil
- 1 pint blueberries
- 1 butternut squash
- 1 cantaloupe
- 1 small bag baby carrots
- 1 bag carrots
- 1 head cauliflower
- 2 pints cherry tomatoes
- 1 cup dried cranberries
- 1 English cucumber
- 1 head garlic
- 2-inch piece fresh ginger
- 1 bunch grapes
- 2 cups green beans
- 3 scallions
- 2 kiwis
- 2 leeks
- 2 lemons
- 3 limes
- 2 mangoes
- 1 pound button or white mushrooms
- 3 oranges
- 2 red onions
- 1 bunch fresh parsley
- 6 peaches
- 2 red bell peppers
- 1 potato
- 1 small bag new potatoes
- 3 ounces golden raisins
- 1 pint raspberries
- 3 stalks rhubarb
- 1 large bag baby spinach leaves

- 4 tomatoes
- 1 yellow bell pepper
- 2 green zucchini

Whole Grains

- 1 box or bag brown rice
- 1 loaf multigrain bread
- 1 bag large-flake oatmeal
- 1 box or bag dried quinoa
- 1 box organic puffed quinoa
- 1 bag whole-grain bagels

Nuts, Seeds, and Oils

Note: Some supermarkets have a bulk-goods section where you can scoop dried goods such as nuts and seeds out of bins in the quantities you want.

- 4 ounces almonds
- 1 jar natural nut butter (almond butter or your choice)
- 1 bag shredded, unsweetened coconut
- 1 ounce flaxseed
- 1 bottle extra-virgin olive oil
- 3 ½ ounces pecan halves
- 1 bottle sesame oil
- 1 ounce sesame seeds
- 5 ounces sunflower seeds

Pantry Items

- 1 bottle apple cider vinegar
- 1 jar unsweetened apple sauce
- 1 box baking soda
- 1 jar ground or cracked black pepper

- 1 jar brown rice syrup
- 1 bar 70 percent dark chocolate
- 1 jar ground cinnamon
- 1 container unsweetened cocoa powder
- 1 box cornstarch
- 1 jar Thai red curry paste
- 1 jar Dijon mustard
- 1 bottle honey
- 1 bottle maple syrup
- 8 ounces freshly squeezed orange juice
- 1 can pineapple juice
- 1 jar dried thyme
- 1 bottle pure vanilla extract

WEEK 2 SHOPPING LIST

Proteins and Dairy

- 8 ounces almond milk
- 5 (4-ounce) skinless, boneless chicken breasts
- 1 can chickpeas
- 1 quart coconut milk
- 1 container nonfat cottage cheese
- 1 dozen eggs
- 1 container low-sodium feta
- 10-ounce flank steak
- 5 (5-ounce) boneless pork chops, trimmed of visible fat
- 2 pounds boneless pork loin
- 5 ounces tilapia
- 1 can low-sodium, water-packed canned tuna
- 2 (16-ounce) containers nonfat or low-fat plain Greek yogurt

Veggies and Fruit

- 13 apples
- 3 ounces dried apricots
- 1½ ounces arugula
- 1 avocado
- 9 bananas
- 4 heads broccoli
- 6 ounces Brussels sprouts
- 1 butternut squash
- 1 cabbage
- 1 cantaloupe
- 2 carrots
- 1 head celery
- 1 pound cherries
- 1 pint cherry tomatoes
- 2 fennel bulbs
- 1 head garlic
- 1-inch piece fresh ginger root
- 1 grapefruit
- 10½ ounces green beans
- 1 honeydew melon
- 2 lemons
- 3 white or yellow onions
- 1 red onion
- 1 orange
- 1 bunch fresh parsley
- 3 potatoes
- 1 bunch red grapes
- 2 red bell peppers
- 1 bunch fresh rosemary
- 3 scallions
- 1 bag baby spinach
- 3 pints strawberries
- 2 sweet potatoes

- 1 bunch fresh thyme
- 3 tomatoes
- 1 seedless watermelon
- 1 green zucchini

Whole Grains

- 1 container whole-wheat breadcrumbs
- 12 ounces dry whole-wheat couscous
- 1 bag whole-wheat English muffins
- 1 bag rolled oats
- 1 box whole-wheat penne
- 2 ounces quinoa
- 1 bag brown rice
- 1 bag multigrain tortillas

Nuts, Seeds, and Oils

- 1 jar natural almond butter
- 2 ounces almonds
- 1 bottle extra-virgin olive oil
- 1 cup pecans
- 1 cup roasted sunflower seeds

Pantry Items

- 1 can unsweetened apple juice
- 1 jar ground or cracked black pepper
- 1 carton low-fat, low-sodium chicken broth
- 10 ounces 70 percent dark chocolate
- 1 jar ground cinnamon
- 1 can light coconut milk
- 1 jar curry powder
- 1 jar Dijon mustard

- 1 jar fennel seeds
- 1 jar honey
- 1 bottle maple syrup
- 1 whole nutmeg or 1 jar ground nutmeg
- 1½ ounces raisins
- 1 bottle pure vanilla extract
- 4 quarts low-sodium vegetable stock

CHAPTER FIVE

Clean Cooking

If your refrigerator and pantry are bursting with glorious produce, lean meats, and whole grains waiting to be made into clean meals, you want to cook them right, without adding fat or salt. On the Clean Eating plan, cooking cleanly is as important as shopping cleanly—you can undo all the goodness of a sweet onion if you coat it with white flour and deep-fry it in oil. Fortunately, there are many wonderful ways to prepare and season your Clean Eating meals that help retain all the value of the ingredients. Cooking cleanly might end up being the most fun you've ever had in your kitchen!

PREPARATION TECHNIQUES

Once you bring all that lovely clean food home, it can be overwhelming to think about how you're going to prepare your meals. You don't need to have a chef's kitchen or buy a ton of expensive gadgets to do the job, but it helps to have a few tools and some basic equipment that can make your time well spent and pleasant. Some items that make clean cooking easier are:

- Blender
- Casserole dishes
- Cast-iron skillet
- Citrus juicer
- Citrus zester
- Electric hand mixer
- Food processor
- Good-quality knives
- Grater
- Mandoline slicer
- Measuring cups for dry and liquid ingredients
- Nonstick bakeware
- Nonstick pans
- Nonstick skillet with raised grill ridges
- Pepper grinder
- Set of nesting bowls
- Slow cooker
- Storage containers
- Vegetable peeler

You'll be spending more time in the kitchen when you eat cleanly, so it's a good idea to work efficiently whenever possible. Right when you get home from the supermarket, take the time to process your fresh foods so they're easy to use and take up less space in the fridge. Wash, trim, and cut up the produce and put it in see-through stackable containers marked with dates. Trim all the visible fat from your meats and peel the skin off poultry, then put the meat in well-sealed freezer bags until you are ready to use it.

Quick is best when cooking your food because you can lose nutritional content when you cook your food to death. Be aware of what happens to your food as you prepare it, and tailor the technique to the ingredient. For example, boiling fresh green beans until they're grayish and limp will completely remove all the nutritional value and make them unpalatable, but cooking tomatoes actually makes them more nutritious.

Prepare your meals using healthful cooking methods. Some cooking techniques can add calories and fat while leaching out valuable nutrients, but there are better techniques for almost every recipe. Don't panic—some of the best methods are the simplest and most common. You don't have to be a chef to eat cleanly. Better yet, the best clean cooking techniques preserve and enhance the flavor of the ingredients so your finished dish is delicious as well as healthful. Here are some tips for how to cook cleanly.

- **Baking:** This method is usually associated with desserts and bread, but it's also an extremely effective way to cook meats, poultry, fish, and vegetables. Baking doesn't require added fat, and while baking you can either cover your food or leave it uncovered, depending on the recipe.
- **Blanching:** This method, briefly boiling vegetables, takes a little more attention because it's very easy to over-blanch your vegetables, robbing them of nutrients, color, and flavor. To blanch, bring a pot of water to a rolling boil and then drop the heat a little. Add your vegetables and stir to cover them completely with the water. Watch them carefully and test them frequently; drain them when they're tender but still crisp. For veggies that you'll be eating cold, immediately plunge the drained items into a large bowl of ice water to stop the cooking process and chill them quickly.
- **Braising:** You may have made stew in the oven without realizing that you're braising your food. There's a little fat involved in this technique: the meat or poultry is browned in a pan in just a bit of oil or butter before it's put in the oven with a cooking liquid like stock or water. The best sauces can be made from the liquid left over after braising.

- **Broiling:** Broiling is similar to grilling, except it's done in the oven, where the heat source is above the food rather than below it. Broiling should be done in a two-part pan that's slotted on top so fat drains into the drip pan below. Broiling is good for fish, thinner cuts of meat, and vegetables.
- **Grilling:** Grilling is a wonderful way to cook vegetables, poultry, meats, seafood, fish, vegetables, and even fruit. You may have read recently that charring can produce carcinogens, so don't grill everything you eat every day. But definitely use your grill—it adds flavor while allowing fat to drip away.
- **Poaching:** Many home cooks don't poach their food, except perhaps their morning eggs. Poaching is a lovely, gentle way to cook chicken and fish, because it lends tenderness and infuses the flavor of the poaching liquid (broth, fruit or vegetable juice, or wine) and herbs, and there's no fat added.
- **Roasting:** Roasting is very similar to baking, except that it's done at higher temperatures. It's an excellent technique for poultry, meats, and vegetables. Root vegetables intensify their flavors and sweetness when tossed in a little extra-virgin olive oil and roasted in the oven until tender. Make sure you put a drip rack in the roasting pan, particularly for chicken and turkey, so your food doesn't sit in the dripping fat.
- **Sautéing:** This is a quick way to cook small pieces of food, and it can be healthful, depending on how much oil you use. If your ingredients don't need to be browned, you can actually use a splash of water instead to sauté in a good-quality nonstick pan.
- **Steaming:** This preparation technique is quick and extremely healthful because you're cooking your food in hot steam and nothing else. Two-piece steamer pots are inexpensive and easy to find, or you can use a perforated steamer basket in a pot of gently simmering water. If you want to add flavorings such as herbs or citrus, you can actually put those in the water. Steaming is good for vegetables, fish, seafood, and poultry.
- **Stir-frying:** This technique is fun and quick—toss your ingredients in the skillet and you'll end up with bright, delicious results. This traditional Asian cooking style can be done in a wok or very large nonstick pan with a little water, good oil, or broth. Make sure to cut your ingredients into small pieces, and add delicate items such as snow peas or bok choy at the very end.

CLEAN SPICES AND HERBS: HOW TO ADD FLAVOR

Most of the ingredients used to add flavor to conventional recipes—salt, sugar, sauces, gravies, etc.—aren't part of the Clean Eating plan. Instead, add fresh herbs to make your dishes shine. Herbs are a spectacular way to make food tasty, and they have the added benefit of being good for you. There are hundreds of herbs for cooking, although some are difficult to find outside of specialty food stores. However, there are many common herbs that can be used in Clean Eating recipes.

- **Basil:** Basil is known for its distinctive, almost licorice-like flavor, and is often used in Mediterranean-style dishes featuring tomatoes or peppers. Basil is perfect for sauces, pesto, dressings, and soups, or paired with chicken or fish. The lovely green leaves of this herb are packed with antioxidants, potassium, and vitamins A and K. Buy it fresh for maximum flavor; it's also available dried. Try growing basil at home if you have a nice sunny windowsill inside, or in a sunny patch of your yard in warm weather.

- **Black peppercorn:** Peppercorn is the most commonly used spice in the world and is valued for the heat it brings to any dish. When dried, these tiny fruits are hard and black, and can be ground, crushed, or cracked easily. Green peppercorns, available dried or pickled, are milder and perfect for pickling and sauces. A touch of black pepper in a dish will stimulate your taste buds and cause your stomach to produce hydrochloric acid, which improves the digestive process. The outer layer of black peppercorns is also known to help break down fat cells.

- **Chili powder:** This hot spice is a staple in many dishes from South America, India, and Thailand. Chili powder comes from chilies, a member of the nightshade family. This spice gets its fire from capsaicin, which can reduce the pain of arthritis and inflammation. Chili powder is also a very heart-friendly addition to any dish, and has been found to reduce cholesterol in the blood while boosting immunity.

- **Cinnamon:** There's nothing quite as comforting as the scent of cinnamon in the air while desserts bake or oatmeal cooks. Cinnamon has been used for centuries as medicine for an assortment of ailments. Recent studies have shown that cinnamon might help lower blood sugar levels and reduce bad cholesterol. A compound called cinnamaldehyde can prevent the clumping of blood platelets, which helps reduce the risk of heart problems. (Merali-Ebrahim 2013).

- **Cloves:** This warmly flavored spice is the dried bud of an Indonesian flower, and is a wonderful addition to desserts, chili, and soups. You might not know that cloves are often used in dentistry because their oil is an antibacterial and mild anesthetic. Cloves are nutrient-dense; they are a wonderful source of manganese, omega-3 fatty acids (see the glossary), fiber, calcium, and vitamins C and K. Cloves also contain a substance called eugenol, which has been shown to help reduce toxicity from pollutants.

- **Coriander/cilantro:** Coriander seeds are often found in Middle Eastern cuisine and have a lovely citrus-like flavor and scent. These fragrant seeds are very effective for lowering blood sugar as well as for raising good cholesterol levels while decreasing bad cholesterol. Cilantro, the fresh, green leaves of the coriander plant, has a different kind of citrusy flavor. It can help improve bone health with its high vitamin K content. Both parts of this plant can be used in salsas, curries, soups, and dishes that have a spicy heat.

- **Cumin:** This spice can be used either ground or as whole seeds, and is quite popular in Middle Eastern, Indian, and Mexican dishes because of its almost peppery, citrusy taste. Cumin is a great source of iron, calcium, and manganese, as well as powerful antioxidants. It has been found to stabilize blood sugar levels, boost the immune system, and reduce the risk of ulcers and certain types of cancer (Ebeling and Geary 2012).

- **Dill:** The feathery leaves of this delicate-looking plant give dill pickles their distinctive, strong aroma and flavor. It's used fresh or dry in cuisines from Russia to Germany to Scandinavia, and all the way to Africa. Dill is traditionally found in fish dishes and dressings, but it can be used delectably in other recipes. It's a great source of calcium, which can help promote bone health.

- **Ginger:** Ginger can be used either in its fresh, bulbous, tan-colored form for a hot, sweet flavor, or dried and ground for a mellower effect. For centuries, this aromatic, spicy root has been used as a remedy for stomach problems such as nausea, and it's still a popular natural treatment for motion sickness and pregnancy-related stomach upsets. Ginger has also been linked to treating cancer in recent studies (University of Minnesota 2003). It also contains gingerols, which can help reduce the pain associated with arthritis as well as muscle and joint pain.

- **Nutmeg:** The best way to use nutmeg is to grate it fresh from the seed whenever you need it. This spice partners well with almost any other ingredient, from vegetables to cheeses, and even works in creamy rice pudding desserts. Nutmeg is very rich in nutrients and is a great source of vitamins A and C, calcium, potassium, and magnesium. This spice can be an effective treatment for stomach issues, and is considered to be an anti-inflammatory that can fight damaging bacteria.
- **Oregano:** Oregano is commonly used in Italian dishes, and it can be used with tasty results in soups, meat dishes, dressings, and sauces. This sweet herb, used fresh or dry, is a good source of fiber, calcium, iron, and omega-3 fatty acids. Oregano can be a very effective treatment for many types of infections because it has both antibacterial and antifungal properties.
- **Rosemary:** Rosemary has a strong pine-like flavor and scent, and is used both fresh and dried in many Mediterranean dishes. This herb is very common in meat, fish, and chicken entrées, as well as in stews and soups. Fresh rosemary is fabulous when infused into olive oil or vinegar. Rosemary doesn't just add taste to food; it's also very beneficial to your body. It can help with digestion, boost the immune system, improve memory, and stop inflammation.
- **Tarragon:** This herb has a delightful, sweet licorice-like taste that's beautiful with fish, chicken, sauces, salads, egg dishes, dips, and even some desserts. This herb is very popular in French cuisine and can be used fresh or dried. Tarragon has been used for centuries to treat many ailments, such as toothaches, poor appetite, and digestive problems.
- **Thyme:** Thyme has a fresh, lemony, minty flavor that's a favorite of many cooks and cultures. It can be added fresh or dried to almost any other ingredient, including fruit and eggs, to enhance the taste. Thyme is packed full of antioxidants, which can boost immunity, slow the signs of aging, reduce the risk of cancer, and improve memory. It's also extremely effective against most kinds of inflammation.
- **Turmeric:** Turmeric has a lovely, bright yellow color and is often used in place of much more expensive saffron. It's found extensively in Indian dishes, egg recipes, sauces, and fish dishes. Turmeric is the main spice in curry powder, and has been used as a folk remedy for heartburn and arthritis, and to help with weight lost. Recent studies have shown that turmeric might slow the progression of Alzheimer's disease and stop the spread and reproduction of some cancer cells.

FLOUR SUBSTITUTION GUIDE

One of the ingredients that you should avoid on the Clean Eating plan is refined wheat flour, which includes white (bleached or unbleached) all-purpose, cake, bread, pastry, and even some whole-wheat variations. Whole grains are packed with fiber, minerals, vitamins, and phytonutrients that are lost when their bran and germ are removed and the stripped-down grains are pulverized into powder. This starchy stuff is digested faster than whole-grain flour, leading to blood-sugar spikes and inflammation. Refined flour has also been linked to gastrointestinal issues, bone loss, and obesity.

Whole grain also refers to products that include gluten such as wheat, rye, barley, and other cereal grains. Oats can be found in gluten-free form, but unless otherwise labeled, assume that your oatmeal has gluten in it. There are a lot of whole-grain and non-grain flours that can be used instead of refined products with great success in your Clean Eating recipes. However, the finished products won't be exactly like those you get with traditional refined flour. For example, breads made with gluten-free flours are often more cake-like and denser in texture, and pastas made with brown rice and spelt flours can get gluey more easily than regular pasta. Enjoy the interesting differences!

- **Almond flour:** This nutrition-packed flour of very finely ground blanched almonds is a staple in many gluten-free and Paleo kitchens. It's a great source of vitamins, protein, calcium, iron, and zinc. When baking with almond flour, you can simply replace refined flour 1:1, but the finished product might be a bit crumbly if you don't add a couple more eggs.
- **Amaranth:** This flour isn't usually used by itself in recipes, but it's a lovely addition for the nutty, slightly sweet, malty taste it gives to cereals, pancakes, breads, and muffins.
- **Arrowroot starch and tapioca starch:** The flours ground from these tubers do contain simple carbohydrates, so use them infrequently. Arrowroot and tapioca starch impart a lovely, light texture to baked items and are very effective thickening agents for sauces and soups.
- **Brown rice flour:** This fine-textured flour is usually mixed with other flours. It's wonderful in gravy or sauces and has all the nutrition of unpolished brown rice.
- **Buckwheat flour:** Even though its name includes the word *wheat*, buckwheat is neither a kind of wheat nor a grass (as wheat is). Buckwheat flour can be a bit of an acquired taste because it has a very strong, earthy flavor;

it's best when blended with other flours. The base of soba noodles, this flour is also commonly used in pancakes, blintzes, and waffles.

- **Coconut flour:** Coconut flour takes a little getting used to because it soaks up liquid like a sponge. It takes very little coconut flour to substitute for wheat flour—about a quarter cup for one cup of wheat flour. This flour is made by grinding up coconut pulp after the milk has been squeezed out.

- **Cornmeal:** When taking a sunshine-bright, crunchy loaf of Clean Eating cornbread out of the oven, you'll appreciate this flour. Cornmeal is usually used for breads and tortillas, and as polenta and hot cereal.

- **Kamut flour:** Flour made from this ancient grain has a lovely, pale golden color and a somewhat buttery flavor. It's related to wheat but doesn't contain gluten, so many people with wheat sensitivities can eat baked products made with kamut flour.

- **Millet flour:** This underutilized grain is usually associated with birdseed rather than baking. It's the only grain that doesn't contain phytic acid (which blocks minerals in the body), so it can be digested very easily. Millet is high in iron, protein, and calcium. The flour can be used in many different recipes, from cereals to breads.

- **Oat flour (can contain gluten):** You probably have oatmeal in your kitchen, so oat flour will taste familiar. It's very high in protein and is a wonderful choice for pancakes, smoothies, muffins, and other baked items.

- **Quinoa flour:** Clean Eating enthusiasts tend to eat a lot of quinoa, but mostly in the form of hot cereal or as a tasty substitute for rice. But its flour has the same high-protein content and makes a great addition to recipes that are based on other flours.

- **Spelt flour:** Spelt is an ancient type of wheat that's high in fiber and protein, including gluten. If you don't have a gluten allergy, spelt is easier to digest than wheat flour. Its flour is quite nutty in flavor, so it goes well with raisins and other dried fruits. You can use spelt flour much as you would whole-wheat flour in most recipes, adding less liquid than you do with white flour. If you're making bread with spelt flour, don't over-knead the dough, or it will get very stretchy and the bread will be tough.

- **Teff flour:** This less-familiar flour can be hard to find outside health food stores, but it's a great choice for pancakes or waffles, baked items, and breads. It has a wonderful, malty, sweetish taste.

- **Whole-wheat flour (contains gluten):** This flour is made from the entire wheat berry, which gives it a lovely texture, robust flavor, and all the nutrition that wheat has to offer. If you make a recipe with whole-wheat flour alone, you'll get a very dense final product, so blend it with other flours if you're looking for a lighter texture.

Flour Substitution Chart

1 CUP WHITE WHEAT FLOUR EQUALS:	
ALMOND FLOUR	1 CUP
AMARANTH FLOUR	⅞ CUP
ARROWROOT STARCH/TAPIOCA STARCH	¾ CUP
BROWN RICE FLOUR	⅞ CUP
BUCKWHEAT FLOUR	⅞ CUP
COCONUT FLOUR	¼ CUP
CORNMEAL	1 CUP
KAMUT FLOUR	1 CUP
MILLET FLOUR	¾ CUP
OAT FLOUR	1 CUP
QUINOA FLOUR	1 CUP
SPELT FLOUR	1 CUP
WHOLE-WHEAT FLOUR	1 CUP

GUIDE TO GRAINS AND GRAIN-LIKE SEEDS

Whole grains (and a few grain-like seeds) are one of the cornerstones of the Clean Eating plan for good reason: these unrefined foods still have their bran and germ—which contain the main nutritional elements of grain, including fiber. You might not have experimented with the variety of whole grains out there, so you might not realize how delicious they taste and how easy they are to prepare. Note: Store uncooked grains out of direct sunlight in well-sealed containers. Put them in the freezer if you don't plan to use them for three months or longer.

When you're eating cleanly, you also want to take whole grains out of the side dish and casserole category and use them throughout the day in many different ways. For example, you can combine them in a lovely textured pilaf that would be great for any meal. Other possibilities include:

- **Breakfast:** You can make almost any grain into a nice porridge or sprinkle some of the smaller ones into an energy-packed smoothie. Whole grains are also wonderful in homemade granola or stirred into scrambled eggs or a frittata. Keep in mind that breakfast can be anything you want it to be: try a wheat berry salad tossed with an assortment of chopped vegetables.
- **Lunch:** Grains are a great salad base and go with any combination of ingredients. They can also be wonderful soup stars—in hearty beef and barley soup or chicken and wild rice soup, for instance. Try spooning cooked grains into lettuce wraps with some spicy chicken or beef.
- **Dinner:** Grains have long been a standard side dish in many homes, but they can also be perfect in main dishes such as casseroles and stews. You can also toss whole grains with some shredded meat to make stuffing for peppers or squash.
- **Desserts and snacks:** Grains can be sprinkled on yogurt, made into creamy puddings, puffed for munching, made into snack bars, and used in tasty crumbles over stewed fruit.

Clean Eating Whole Grain Guide

GRAIN	FACTS	USES	COOKING TIME
Amaranth	Not a true grain; the seed of a plant related to beets. Great source of fiber, calcium, iron, magnesium, protein, vitamins, and the amino acid lysine. Boosts immunity, reduces cholesterol levels, and lowers blood pressure.	Baking, hot cereal, popping, side dishes, soups	Quick (less than 10 minutes)
Barley (contains gluten)	Great source of fiber, selenium, phosphorus, and copper. Can help lower cholesterol, promote digestive health, and reduce the risk of cardiovascular disease and diabetes.	Hot cereal, salads, side dishes, soups	Medium (10 to 40 minutes)
Buckwheat	Not a true grain; the seed of a plant related to rhubarb and sorrel. Nearly a complete protein, rich in flavonoids (see the glossary), manganese, and fiber. Can reduce the risk of cardiovascular disease and diabetes; helps prevent gallstones.	Baking, hot cereal, salads, side dishes	Medium (10 to 40 minutes)
Bulgur (contains gluten)	Whole wheat kernels that have been boiled, dried, and cracked. High in fiber, iron, protein, and vitamin B_6. Promotes healthy digestion, boosts the immune system, and increases energy.	Casseroles, chili, hot cereal, salads, side dishes	Quick (less than 10 minutes)

GRAIN	FACTS	USES	COOKING TIME
Corn	Corn can be used as cornmeal, cornstarch, or even as popcorn. Cornmeal is dried corn kernels that have been ground; available in different textures. Cornstarch is corn that has been ground down to a powdery texture. Popcorn is a corn variety that is dried. All kinds of corn products are very rich in antioxidants. Can reduce the risk of certain cancers and heart disease.	Baking, hot cereal, popping, side dishes	Medium (10 to 40 minutes)
Freekeh (contains gluten)	Young wheat that has been picked while green. Higher in protein, fiber, vitamins, and minerals than other grains, and has a lower glycemic index (see the glossary). Supports digestion, promotes healthy eyes, and facilitates weight loss.	Casseroles, hot cereal, pudding, side dishes, soups	Medium (10 to 40 minutes)
Millet	A mild-flavored grain most often used as birdseed. Gluten-free. High in manganese, magnesium, niacin, and phosphorous. Very heart-friendly, lowers the risk of diabetes, promotes cell repair, and reduces the risk of breast cancer.	Casseroles, hot cereal, side dishes, smoothies	Quick (less than 10 minutes)

GRAIN	FACTS	USES	COOKING TIME
Oats, large-flake (can contain gluten)	Contains the fiber beta-glucan, vitamins, protein, minerals, and more soluble fiber than any other grain. Helps lower cholesterol, reduce the risk of heart disease, protect blood vessels, and stabilize blood sugar. Oats can be gluten-free and can be called "large flake" (same as rolled or old-fashioned) or "quick-cooking." Large-flake oats are whole grains that have been steamed and rolled flat. Quick-cooking oats are large-flake oats that have been chopped into smaller pieces.	Baking, hot cereal, meatloaf filler	Quick (less than 10 minutes); very quick for quick-cooking oats (less than 5 minutes)
Oats, steel-cut (can contain gluten)	A very filling grain that is the inner part of the oat kernel. This whole groat is then cut into different size pieces. This oat product has not been steamed. Contains the fiber beta-glucan, vitamins, protein, and minerals. Helps lower cholesterol, protect blood vessels, and stabilize blood sugar.	Hot cereal, salads	Medium (10 to 40 minutes)

GRAIN	FACTS	USES	COOKING TIME
Quinoa	Not a true grain; the seed of a plant related to beets and spinach. Many different colors, lovely nutty flavor. A complete protein and extremely high in iron. Helps lower cholesterol levels. Reduces the risk of cardiovascular disease, diabetes, and breast cancer.	Casseroles, hot cereal, main dishes, salads, side dishes, soups	Quick (less than 10 minutes)
Rice, brown	Great source of manganese, fiber, selenium, iron, and other nutrients. Can boost energy, help with weight loss, promote digestive health, and lower cholesterol.	Casseroles, hot cereal, main dishes, side dishes	Medium (10 to 40 minutes)
Rice, wild	The seed of a marsh-grass plant. Twice the protein and fiber of brown rice. Gluten-free and very rich in antioxidants. Can help boost immunity, heart health, and energy levels.	Hot cereal, main dishes, salads, side dishes	Long (more than 40 minutes)
Rye berries (contains gluten)	A grain with rich taste and hearty texture. Very high in fiber, manganese, and phosphorous. Can help promote weight loss, prevent gallstones, and lower the risk of type 2 diabetes.	Baking, casseroles, salads, soups	Long (more than 40 minutes)

GRAIN	FACTS	USES	COOKING TIME
Spelt	A type of wheat that is an ancient ancestor of modern-day wheat. Rich, almost nutty taste. Very high in manganese, fiber, phosphorous, protein, and copper. Helps lower cholesterol levels and reduces the risk of cardiovascular disease, diabetes, and breast cancer.	Baking, hot cereal, salads, side dishes	Long (more than 40 minutes)
Teff	A tiny, nutrient-packed grain that's high in protein, calcium, vitamin C, iron, phosphorus, zinc, B vitamins, and eight amino acids. Can help stabilize blood sugar, facilitate weight control, and promote colon health.	Baking, hot cereal	Medium (10 to 40 minutes)
Wheat berries (contains gluten)	The whole wheat kernel, with its bran, germ, and endosperm. Very high in protein, fiber, vitamin E, and B vitamins. Promotes good digestion, reduces the risk of cardiovascular disease, supports healthy skin, and helps fight obesity.	Main dishes, salads, side dishes	Long (more than 40 minutes)

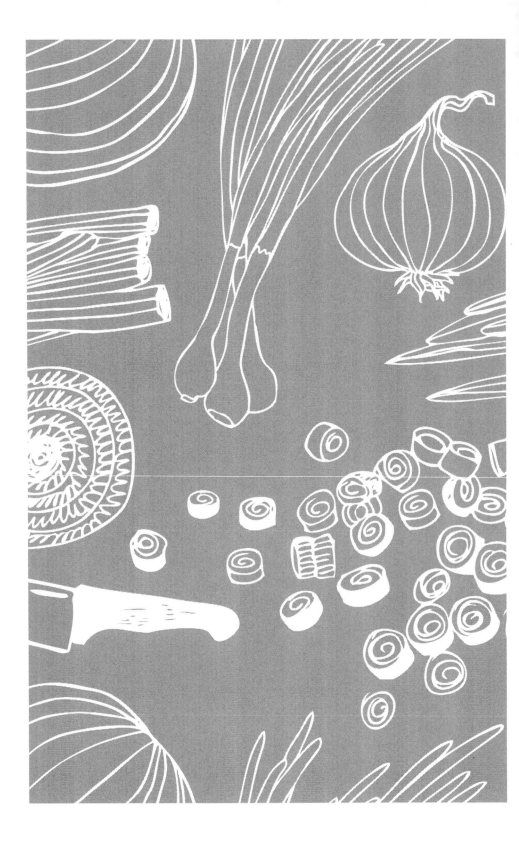

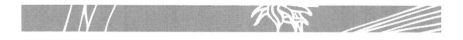

PART TWO

105 Clean Eating Recipes

RECIPE KEY

Each recipe will be labeled with one or more of the following categories right at the beginning so you can pick factors that are important to your meal.

- **Winter:** The main ingredient and/or several of the secondary ingredients are freshest in winter. In North America and other northern hemisphere areas, this would mean December through March.
- **Spring:** The main ingredient and/or several of the secondary ingredients are freshest in spring. In North America and other northern hemisphere areas, this would mean April through June.
- **Summer:** The main ingredient and/or several of the secondary ingredients are freshest in summer. In North America and other northern hemisphere areas, this would mean July and August.
- **Fall:** The main ingredient and/or several of the secondary ingredients are freshest in autumn. In North America and other northern hemisphere areas, this would mean September through November.
- **Any season:** The main ingredient and/or several of the secondary ingredients are equally fresh any time of year.
- **Quick & easy:** This recipe takes less than thirty minutes to prepare and cook. This doesn't include marinating time for meats or freezing time for ice creams or sorbets.
- **Low-fat:** For every 100 calories, this dish has 3 grams of fat or less.
- **Low-sodium:** This recipe has 140 mg of sodium or less per serving.
- **High protein:** This recipe has a protein content that is 25 to 35 percent of the calories of the dish.
- **Budget-friendly:** The ingredients in this dish are readily available and reasonably priced, especially when in season.
- **Super food:** This recipe contains at least one Clean Eating super food ingredient with particularly notable nutritional content and health benefits.

CHAPTER SIX

Smoothies

Chia Berry Smoothie

SERVES 2

- LATE SUMMER/FALL
- QUICK & EASY
- HIGH PROTEIN
- SUPER FOOD

This smoothie won't exactly have a smooth texture, due to the seeds from the berries and the chia seeds (see the glossary). Blackberries and blueberries are in season at roughly the same time of year, so enjoy this smoothie in late summer and fall for the best flavor.

1 CUP BLACKBERRIES
1 CUP BLUEBERRIES
2 TABLESPOONS CHIA SEEDS
1 TEASPOON PURE VANILLA EXTRACT
1½ CUPS UNSWEETENED COCONUT MILK
1 SCOOP UNFLAVORED OR VANILLA PROTEIN POWDER
    (SEE THE GLOSSARY)

In a blender, process all the ingredients until smooth. Serve in a tall glass.

Green Energy Smoothie

SERVES 2

- ANY SEASON
- QUICK & EASY
- HIGH PROTEIN
- SUPER FOOD

The "green" in this smoothie is an ingredient you may never have heard of before: spirulina. Spirulina is a blue-green algae that grows in warm, fresh water. Sound scary? Don't worry—in this smoothie you won't even know it's there, except for the fun color. Spirulina has been used for centuries as a highly nutritious food source by many cultures. It can boost your immune system, balance blood pressure, and lower cholesterol, and it contains more protein than red meat does. You can find it in health food stores.

1 BANANA

1 CUP ALMOND MILK

½ CUP LOW-FAT PLAIN YOGURT

½ CUP UNSWEETENED APPLESAUCE

4 TABLESPOONS LARGE-FLAKE OATMEAL

1 TEASPOON SPIRULINA POWDER

1 TEASPOON PURE VANILLA EXTRACT

In a blender, process all the ingredients until smooth. If you want a thicker smoothie, add a few ice cubes. Serve in a tall glass.

Nutty Berry Smoothie

SERVES 2

- SPRING
- QUICK & EASY
- HIGH PROTEIN

Strawberries impart a lovely sweetness to this tasty drink. Only eight strawberries provide about 140 percent of the recommended daily amount (RDA) of vitamin C, so this smoothie is a wonderful way to start your day. The hemp will add a nutty taste that enhances the cashews.

2 CUPS SLICED STRAWBERRIES

2 TABLESPOONS CHOPPED CASHEWS

1 TABLESPOON SUNFLOWER SEEDS

1 TABLESPOON HEMP SEEDS

1 CUP VANILLA ALMOND MILK

In a blender, process all the ingredients until smooth. Serve in a tall glass.

Pear Green Tea Smoothie

SERVES 2

- FALL
- QUICK & EASY
- SUPER FOOD

In order to get the most benefit from your green tea smoothie, try to find Matcha green tea powder—it is of the highest quality. This powder is from Japan, where it has been consumed for more than one thousand years. Green tea is packed with antioxidants, chlorophyll (see the glossary), and fiber.

2 PEARS, CORED AND CHOPPED

2 CUPS COCONUT MILK

2 TABLESPOONS GREEN TEA POWDER, STIRRED INTO 2 TABLESPOONS
   HOT WATER

1½ CUPS ICE CUBES

In a blender, process all the ingredients until smooth. Serve in a tall glass.

Kiwi Spinach Smoothie

SERVES 2

- FALL/WINTER
- QUICK & EASY
- LOW-SODIUM

This smoothie is a fresh, pretty shade of green that will make you feel healthier just holding it. When purchasing the kiwis, try to select ripe fruit to avoid bitterness. Hold the kiwi lightly in your cupped hand and gently squeeze it. There should be a slight give to the skin but not mushiness.

3 KIWIS, PEELED AND CHOPPED

2 PACKED CUPS BABY SPINACH

1 BANANA

½ CUP UNSWEETENED APPLE JUICE

½ CUP COCONUT MILK

1 TEASPOON HONEY

1 CUP ICE CUBES

In a blender, process all the ingredients except the ice cubes. Add the ice cubes and blend until smooth. Serve in a tall glass.

CHAPTER SEVEN

Breakfasts

Melon Breakfast Salad

SERVES 4

- SUMMER
- LOW-FAT
- LOW-SODIUM
- SUPER FOOD

Watermelons are a perennial favorite, but they can be frustrating because it seems like you never know if you have a good one until you cut it open. Look for a uniformly dark green melon that feels quite heavy for its size. Turn it over to make sure the spot where it sat on the ground is yellowish, rather than white or light green; those colors mean that the melon was probably picked too soon and won't be ripe.

½ SEEDLESS WATERMELON, RIND REMOVED AND FLESH
    CUT INTO 1-INCH CHUNKS
¼ CANTALOUPE, PEELED, SEEDED, AND CUT INTO 1-INCH CHUNKS
1 CUP SLICED STRAWBERRIES
1 CUP BLUEBERRIES
½ ENGLISH CUCUMBER, DICED
1 CUP HALVED RED GRAPES
PINCH OF CAYENNE PEPPER
2 TABLESPOONS JULIENNED FRESH MINT LEAVES

In a large bowl, toss all the ingredients together. Let them stand for about 60 minutes, tossing several times. Serve in shallow bowls.

Mediterranean Omelet

SERVES 4

- SUMMER/FALL
- QUICK & EASY
- LOW-SODIUM
- HIGH PROTEIN

The traditional technique for omelet-making is quite complicated, and many professional chefs can't even produce perfect results. This omelet, however, requires no fancy pan work and is very simple to prepare. All you really have to do is let it sit over heat until it's set.

1 TEASPOON EXTRA-VIRGIN OLIVE OIL

2 CUPS EGG WHITES

1 TABLESPOON CHOPPED FRESH BASIL

¼ TEASPOON FRESHLY GROUND BLACK PEPPER

½ TEASPOON MINCED GARLIC

½ CUP CHOPPED YELLOW BELL PEPPER

½ CUP FINELY CHOPPED RED ONION

1 CUP HALVED CHERRY TOMATOES

1. Preheat the oven to broil.

2. In a large ovenproof skillet over medium heat, heat the olive oil.

3. In a medium bowl, thoroughly combine the egg whites, basil, and black pepper. Set aside.

4. Add the garlic and bell pepper to the skillet and sauté until tender and fragrant, about 2 minutes. Add the onions and tomatoes and sauté for another minute.

continued ▶

5. Remove the skillet from the heat and pour in the egg whites. Put the skillet back on the heat and cover it. Cook the omelet for 10 to 12 minutes without stirring, until egg mixture is set.

6. Remove the skillet from the heat and put it under the broiler for about 60 seconds, until the top is lightly browned.

7. Cut the omelet into quarters and transfer the pieces to plates.

Clean Eating Granola

MAKES 20 SERVINGS

- ANY SEASON
- HIGH PROTEIN
- SUPER FOOD

This recipe isn't set in stone; you can add your favorite nuts, seeds, and dried fruit to create your own customized, delicious Clean Eating food. Make sure you keep the foundation elements—oats, coconut, honey, and oil—so your granola has a good base and holds together well.

6 CUPS LARGE-FLAKE ROLLED OATS

1 CUP SHREDDED UNSWEETENED COCONUT

½ CUP SUNFLOWER SEEDS

½ CUP SLICED ALMONDS

¼ CUP FLAXSEED

¼ CUP HEMP HEARTS (SHELLED HEMP SEEDS) OR SESAME SEEDS

1 TEASPOON GROUND CINNAMON

¼ CUP CANOLA OIL

¼ CUP HONEY

1 CUP DRIED CRANBERRIES

½ CUP GOLDEN RAISINS

1. Preheat the oven to 250°F.

2. Cover 2 baking sheets with foil and set aside.

3. In a large bowl, stir together the oats, coconut, sunflower seeds, almonds, flaxseed, hemp hearts, and cinnamon until well combined; set aside.

4. In a small microwave-safe bowl, whisk together the oil and honey. Heat on low for 30 seconds, until the mixture is warm and combines easily.

continued ▶

5. Add the honey mixture to the dry ingredients and mix everything together with your hands until well combined.

6. Spread the granola onto the prepared baking sheets and bake it, stirring frequently, until the granola is toasted and golden, about 1½ hours.

7. Remove it from the oven and transfer the granola to large bowl. Add the cranberries and raisins and toss to combine.

8. Cool the granola completely and store it in airtight containers; freeze if desired.

Spanakopita Frittata

SERVES 8

- SUMMER/FALL
- HIGH PROTEIN
- SUPER FOOD

Anyone who has enjoyed the buttery, flaky Greek pastries stuffed with spinach and cheese will love this Clean Eating tribute. It's important to use low-sodium feta because traditional feta has about 1,200 mg of sodium per half cup—too much for most people eating cleanly. You can also reduce the amount of feta in the frittata with little effect on the flavor.

1 TEASPOON EXTRA-VIRGIN OLIVE OIL

6 EGG WHITES

2 EGGS

2 CUPS SPINACH

1 TOMATO, SEEDED AND CHOPPED

½ CUP ROASTED, CHOPPED RED BELL PEPPER

½ CUP CRUMBLED LOW-SODIUM FETA

¼ TEASPOON FRESHLY GROUND BLACK PEPPER

1. Preheat the oven to 350°F.

2. Grease a 9-by-13-inch cake pan with the oil and set aside.

3. In a large bowl, thoroughly whisk together the egg whites and eggs. Stir in all the other ingredients until well combined.

4. Pour the egg mixture into the prepared pan. Bake the frittata until just set, 18 to 22 minutes.

5. Remove the pan from the oven and put it on a wire rack. Cool the frittata for about 5 minutes.

6. Loosen the edges of the frittata with a rubber spatula, and cut it into 8 pieces. Slide the spatula under the pieces and lift them onto plates.

Steel-Cut Oatmeal

SERVES 4

- ANY SEASON
- BUDGET-FRIENDLY
- HIGH PROTEIN
- SUPER FOOD

Steel-cut oatmeal can be an acquired taste, especially if you're used to gummy single-serve oatmeal. The texture of this porridge will depend on how long you cook the oats; if you like a chewier texture, follow the recipe as given here. If you want a smoother eating experience, increase the cooking time, adding liquid when required. Or you can cook your porridge overnight in a slow cooker.

3 CUPS STEEL-CUT OATS

4 CUPS WATER

2 CUPS ALMOND MILK

¼ CUP SUNFLOWER SEEDS

1 TABLESPOON GROUND FLAXSEED

1. In a medium saucepan, stir together all the ingredients. Cover the pan and place it over medium-high heat until the mixture starts to simmer.

2. Reduce the heat to low and continue to cook, stirring occasionally, for about 60 minutes, until the oatmeal is chewy but tender.

3. Serve warm with Clean Eating toppings such as dried fruit, nuts, apple-sauce, or fresh berries.

Clean Huevos Rancheros Wraps

SERVES 4

- SUMMER/FALL
- QUICK & EASY
- BUDGET-FRIENDLY
- HIGH PROTEIN
- SUPER FOOD

This is the perfect grab-and-go breakfast or snack for all-day energy. If you're going to eat this on the run, you don't want to end up wearing it, so make sure your eggs are cooked quite dry and the bean mixture is thick. Don't overstuff the wrap, either, or your wrapper won't encase the filling completely.

2 CUPS DRAINED AND RINSED CANNED SODIUM-FREE
    BLACK BEANS
4 SCALLIONS, SLICED
½ RED BELL PEPPER, CUT INTO THIN STRIPS
2 TOMATOES, SEEDED AND CHOPPED
1 TEASPOON MINCED GARLIC
1 TEASPOON GROUND CUMIN
1 TEASPOON EXTRA-VIRGIN OLIVE OIL
8 EGG WHITES
8 MULTIGRAIN SANDWICH WRAPS OR TORTILLAS
4 TABLESPOONS NONFAT PLAIN GREEK YOGURT
SPLASH OF HOT SAUCE (OPTIONAL)

1. Heat a large skillet over medium-high heat.

2. Add the beans, scallions, red pepper, tomatoes, garlic, and cumin and cook, stirring occasionally, for about 4 minutes. With the back of a wooden spoon, mash the beans a little. Remove the pan from the heat and set aside.

continued ▶

3. Grease a small skillet with the oil and scramble the egg whites over medium heat until dry but not browned.

4. Scoop ⅛ of the eggs onto each wrapper and top with ⅛ of the bean mixture plus ½ tablespoon of yogurt.

5. Splash a little hot sauce on each portion (if using) and roll the wraps up neatly.

6. Serve 2 wraps per person.

Baked Citrus French Toast

SERVES 4

- ANY SEASON
- HIGH PROTEIN
- SUPER FOOD

This is a decadent breakfast suitable for lazy mornings and special occasions. You won't be cooking the toast in butter on top of the stove, but baking it to avoid adding fat. But you won't lose any flavor! You can even make a double batch and freeze half of it, then pop the toasts in the toaster oven or microwave when you're ready to eat them.

EXTRA-VIRGIN OLIVE OIL FOR THE BAKING SHEET

4 EGG WHITES

½ CUP ALMOND MILK

1 TEASPOON PURE VANILLA EXTRACT

FRESH JUICE AND ZEST OF 1 ORANGE

1 TEASPOON LEMON ZEST

PINCH OF GROUND CINNAMON

8 SLICES MULTIGRAIN BREAD

FRESH BERRIES FOR TOPPING (OPTIONAL)

1. Preheat the oven to 450°F.

2. Cover a baking sheet with foil and coat it lightly with the oil. Set aside.

3. In a medium bowl, whisk the egg whites, almond milk, vanilla, orange juice and zest, lemon zest, and cinnamon until well blended.

4. Lightly dredge each bread slice in the egg mixture on both sides and shake off any excess liquid.

5. Place the slices side by side on the baking sheet.

6. Bake for 5 minutes or until the toast is golden, then turn the toast over and bake for 5 more minutes.

7. Serve warm, either plain or with fresh berries (if using).

Butternut Squash Pancakes

SERVES 6

- FALL/WINTER
- HIGH PROTEIN
- BUDGET-FRIENDLY
- SUPER FOOD

This is a lovely, hearty breakfast choice. Squash might seem like a strange ingredient for pancakes, but its sweetness works very well with the warm spices. In contrast to other winter squashes, butternut squash is perfect for this recipe, because its firm, finely textured flesh isn't stringy. Look for a deep orange color that indicates the squash is ripe and sweet.

1½ CUPS WHOLE-WHEAT FLOUR

½ CUP ALMOND FLOUR

2 TEASPOONS BAKING POWDER

½ TEASPOON GROUND CINNAMON

½ TEASPOON GROUND NUTMEG

½ TEASPOON GROUND GINGER

PINCH OF SEA SALT (OPTIONAL)

1½ CUPS NONFAT MILK

1 CUP COOKED MASHED BUTTERNUT SQUASH

½ CUP EGG WHITES

¼ CUP MAPLE SYRUP

2 TABLESPOONS CANOLA OIL

EXTRA-VIRGIN OLIVE OIL FOR THE SKILLET

FRESH FRUIT FOR TOPPING (OPTIONAL)

1. Into a large bowl, sift together the flours, baking powder, spices, and salt (if using).

2. In a medium bowl, whisk together the milk, cooked squash, egg whites, maple syrup, and canola oil until combined.

3. Add the wet ingredients to the dry ingredients and stir until the batter is just moistened.

4. Lightly coat a large, heavy skillet with the olive oil and heat over medium heat. For each pancake, pour about $\frac{1}{4}$ cup of the batter into the skillet, about 4 pancakes at a time.

5. Cook the pancakes until they bubble on the surface and their edges are firm, about 2 minutes. Turn the pancakes over and cook them about 2 more minutes. Remove the pancakes to a warm plate and cover with a clean dish towel to keep warm. Repeat until all the batter is used up.

6. Serve warm, either plain or with fresh fruit (if using).

Rhubarb Bread Pudding for the Slow Cooker

SERVES 8

- SPRING/EARLY SUMMER
- HIGH PROTEIN
- SUPER FOOD

Although it's often used in fruity dishes such as pies, puddings, and compotes, rhubarb is actually a vegetable. It's very rich in fiber, antioxidants, and vitamins C and K, benefitting your heart, digestion, and immune system. Take care not to eat any part of the large, heart-shaped leaves, as they're very poisonous. Only use the stalks, which can grow to more than 1½ feet long.

EXTRA-VIRGIN OLIVE OIL FOR THE SLOW COOKER

3 CUPS NONFAT MILK

4 EGGS, BEATEN

FRESH JUICE AND ZEST OF 1 ORANGE

½ CUP MAPLE SYRUP

2 TABLESPOONS CORNSTARCH

1 TEASPOON PURE VANILLA EXTRACT

12 SLICES MULTIGRAIN BREAD, CUBED

1 CUP CHOPPED FRESH RHUBARB

1. Oil the bottom and sides of a slow-cooker insert; set aside.

2. In a large bowl, combine the milk, eggs, orange juice and zest, maple syrup, cornstarch, and vanilla. Add the bread and stir to combine. Add the rhubarb and stir.

3. Spoon the bread mixture into the slow cooker. Cover and cook on high heat for 1 hour, then reduce heat to medium-low and cook until the custard is set, about 1 hour.

4. Serve warm.

Buckwheat Crêpes with Strawberries

SERVES 5

- SPRING/SUMMER
- BUDGET-FRIENDLY
- HIGH PROTEIN
- SUPER FOOD

Buckwheat is incredibly beneficial for the cardiovascular system because it's a great source of magnesium. It has also been proven very effective for stabilizing blood sugar. Leftover crêpes can be frozen between sheets of parchment or wax paper.

1½ CUPS NONFAT MILK

3 EGGS

1 TEASPOON EXTRA-VIRGIN OLIVE OIL, PLUS MORE FOR THE SKILLET

1 CUP BUCKWHEAT FLOUR

½ CUP WHOLE-WHEAT FLOUR

2 CUPS SLICED STRAWBERRIES

1. In a large bowl, whisk the milk, eggs, and 1 teaspoon of oil until well combined.

2. Into a medium bowl, sift together the flours. Add the dry ingredients to the wet ingredients and whisk until well combined and very smooth.

3. Allow the batter to rest for at least 2 hours before cooking.

4. Heat a large skillet or crêpe pan over medium-high heat. Lightly coat the bottom of the skillet with oil. Pour about ¼ cup of batter into the skillet. Swirl the pan until the batter completely coats the bottom.

continued ▶

5. Cook the crêpe for about 1 minute, then flip it over. Cook the second side of the crêpe for another minute until lightly browned. Transfer the cooked crêpe to a plate and cover with a clean dish towel to keep warm.

6. Repeat until the batter is used up; you should have about 10 crêpes.

7. Spoon 3 tablespoons of the strawberries onto each crêpe and roll it up. Serve 2 crêpes per plate.

Pumpkin Apple Oatmeal

SERVES 2

- FALL/WINTER
- QUICK & EASY
- SUPER FOOD

Eating this oatmeal is like being wrapped in a warm blanket in front of a crackling fire on a cool autumn day. You can use fresh-cooked or canned pumpkin with the same results, as long as your canned product is simple pumpkin rather than pie filling, which contains a lot of sugar and sodium.

⅔ CUP WATER

⅓ CUP UNSWEETENED APPLE JUICE

2 TABLESPOONS MAPLE SYRUP

4 TABLESPOONS COOKED, MASHED PUMPKIN

¾ CUP QUICK-COOKING ROLLED OATS

¾ TEASPOON GROUND CINNAMON

¼ TEASPOON GROUND NUTMEG

1 APPLE, PEELED, CORED, AND DICED

1. In a medium saucepan over medium-high heat, stir together the water, apple juice, maple syrup, and pumpkin and bring to a boil.

2. In a small bowl, combine the oats and spices; stir into the boiling mixture.

3. Cook, stirring occasionally, for about 10 minutes or until the cereal is the desired consistency. You may add more water during cooking if the oatmeal gets too thick.

4. Stir in the apples and serve immediately.

Pear Cranberry Quinoa Cereal

SERVES 6

- FALL/WINTER
- QUICK & EASY
- HIGH PROTEIN
- SUPER FOOD

Quinoa is a very quick-cooking, nutritious choice for breakfast, made even better when you add chopped pear. This recipe uses pears with the skin on, so it's important to scrub the outside of your fruit thoroughly to remove any contaminants or pesticides. You can peel the pears, but the skin has three to four times the phenolic phytonutrients of the flesh of the fruit. This means powerful antioxidant and anti-inflammatory flavonoid (see the glossary) clout right in your breakfast bowl.

2 CUPS WATER

2 CUPS COCONUT MILK

2 CUPS UNCOOKED QUINOA, WASHED AND PICKED OVER

PINCH OF SEA SALT

3 TABLESPOONS MAPLE SYRUP

2 PEARS, CORED AND DICED

4 TABLESPOONS DRIED CRANBERRIES

1. In a medium saucepan, stir together the water, coconut milk, quinoa, and salt.

2. Cover the pan and cook over medium heat until the mixture boils. Reduce the heat and simmer for about 15 minutes, or until the cereal is the desired consistency. You may add more water during cooking if the cereal gets too thick.

3. Stir in the maple syrup, pears, and cranberries. Serve immediately.

Quick Spinach and Eggs

SERVES 4

- SPRING/SUMMER
- QUICK & EASY
- BUDGET-FRIENDLY
- SUPER FOOD

If you don't have a deep, traditional cast-iron skillet, this recipe is one of the reasons you should invest in one. A real cast-iron skillet cooks the eggs evenly and quickly and browns them perfectly because the iron disperses heat beautifully. You also need less oil when cooking with cast iron, as it has a natural, chemical-free, nonstick quality (unlike other nonstick pans). Plus, this kind of pan actually adds iron to your food.

EXTRA-VIRGIN OLIVE OIL FOR THE SKILLET
1 TEASPOON MINCED GARLIC
8 EGG WHITES
½ CUP COCONUT MILK
1 TEASPOON GROUND NUTMEG
1 PACKED CUP SHREDDED BABY SPINACH
1 SCALLION, SLICED THINLY
FRESHLY GROUND BLACK PEPPER

1. Lightly oil a large skillet and place it over medium-high heat.

2. Add the garlic to the skillet and sauté until fragrant, about 2 minutes.

3. In a medium bowl, thoroughly combine the egg whites, coconut milk, nutmeg, spinach, and scallions. Season with pepper.

4. Pour the egg mixture into the heated skillet and cook until the eggs are cooked through, 3 to 5 minutes.

5. Divide among 3 plates, and serve.

Honey Breakfast Cookies

MAKES 12 BARS

- ANY SEASON
- HIGH PROTEIN
- SUPER FOOD

Sometimes you just need to have a cookie for breakfast. This healthful choice is just as delectable as the prepackaged treats. If you want your cookies to be even higher in protein, you can add a scoop of unsweetened or vanilla protein powder to the dry ingredients. These cookies are perfect for mornings when you're playing sports or need an energy boost before school or work.

1 CUP OLD-FASHIONED ROLLED OATS
¼ CUP SLICED ALMONDS
¼ CUP SUNFLOWER SEEDS
2 TABLESPOONS SESAME SEEDS
2 CUPS UNSWEETENED PUFFED RICE
½ CUP CRANBERRIES
½ CUP CHOPPED GOLDEN RAISINS
½ CUP ALMOND BUTTER
¼ CUP HONEY
1 TEASPOON PURE VANILLA EXTRACT
PINCH OF SEA SALT
EXTRA-VIRGIN OLIVE OIL FOR THE BAKING DISH

1. Preheat the oven to 250°F.

2. Line a large baking sheet with foil. Spread the oats, almonds, sunflower seeds, and sesame seeds on the baking sheet and bake, stirring halfway through, until they're lightly toasted, about 30 minutes.

3. Transfer the oat mixture to a large bowl and add the puffed rice, cranberries, and raisins. Toss to combine.

4. In a small saucepan over medium heat, stir together the almond butter, honey, vanilla, and salt and cook until bubbling. Add the hot mixture to the dry ingredients and stir until well combined.

5. Lightly oil an 8-inch-square baking dish or line it with parchment paper. Spoon the batter into the dish and press it down firmly.

6. Refrigerate the slab until firm, about 3 hours. Cut into 12 portions. Store in an airtight container in the refrigerator.

Simple Egg Wraps

SERVES 2

- ANY SEASON
- QUICK & EASY
- BUDGET-FRIENDLY
- HIGH PROTEIN

There's no fuss or muss with these nutritious wraps, and they can be ready in less than ten minutes. You can use regular yogurt in place of Greek, but it's usually not as thick and luscious. Greek yogurt is also strained, which means it has twice the protein and half the milk sugar (lactose; see the glossary) as regular varieties.

4 EGG WHITES
1 WHOLE EGG
2 TABLESPOONS ALMOND MILK
FRESHLY GROUND BLACK PEPPER
EXTRA-VIRGIN OLIVE OIL FOR THE SKILLET
2 TABLESPOONS NONFAT PLAIN GREEK YOGURT
1 TEASPOON CHOPPED FRESH DILL
2 MULTIGRAIN WRAPS

1. In a small bowl, whisk together the egg whites, egg, and milk. Season with pepper.

2. Lightly oil a large skillet over medium-high heat. Pour the egg mixture into the skillet and cook until set, about 1 minute.

3. Remove the omelet from the skillet, spread with yogurt, and sprinkle with dill.

4. Cut the omelet in half and roll each half in a multigrain wrap. Serve immediately.

CHAPTER EIGHT

Snacks

Creamy Fruit Dip

MAKES 1½ CUPS

- ANY SEASON
- QUICK & EASY
- HIGH PROTEIN
- LOW-SODIUM
- SUPER FOOD

This dip works beautifully any time of year because you can use it with all types of fruit. Almond butter adds a nice flavor, but you could use any nut butter with great results. Almonds are full of antioxidants that can help reduce your risk of cardiovascular disease, and they also help stabilize blood sugar, making them a great weight-loss food.

1 CUP NONFAT PLAIN GREEK YOGURT
½ CUP ALMOND BUTTER
½ TEASPOON PURE VANILLA EXTRACT
ASSORTMENT OF CUT FRUIT

1. In a small bowl, stir together the yogurt, almond butter, and vanilla until well blended.

2. Store the dip in the fridge until you're ready to use it.

3. Serve with the fruit.

Clean Eating Corn Bread

MAKES 16 PIECES

- ■ ANY SEASON
- ■ QUICK & EASY
- ■ BUDGET-FRIENDLY
- ■ LOW-SODIUM
- ■ HIGH PROTEIN

You might think of corn bread as fattening, which it can be when it's full of butter, oil, sugar, or extra ingredients such as bacon and cheese. Even though this is a clean recipe, the bread has all the buttery, sweet goodness of traditional cornbread, enhanced by almond flour.

EXTRA-VIRGIN OLIVE OIL FOR THE BAKING DISH

¾ CUP ALMOND FLOUR

1¼ CUPS CORNMEAL

1 TABLESPOON BAKING POWDER

PINCH OF SEA SALT

2 EGGS

1 CUP SOY MILK

3 TABLESPOONS MAPLE SYRUP

3 TABLESPOONS CANOLA OIL

¼ TEASPOON CHOPPED FRESH JALAPEÑO PEPPER

1. Preheat the oven to 425°F.

2. Spread a thin coating of olive oil on the bottom and sides of an 8-inch-square baking dish.

3. In a large bowl, stir together the almond flour, cornmeal, baking powder, and salt. Make a well in the center of the dry ingredients and add the eggs, soy milk, maple syrup, canola oil, and jalapeño. Mix until the batter is well combined.

4. Spoon the batter into the baking dish. Bake the cornbread for 20 minutes.

5. Cut the cornbread into 2-inch squares and serve warm.

Black Bean Salsa Recipe

SERVES 8

- SUMMER
- QUICK & EASY
- BUDGET-FRIENDLY
- SUPER FOOD

Everyone needs a no-fail salsa recipe to whip together when unexpected company drops in. This recipe is bursting with fresh vegetables and goes perfectly with wraps, baked tortilla chips, grilled meats and fish, brown rice, or quinoa. If you like your salsa fiery, you can add more jalapeño. Either wear plastic gloves when chopping your jalapeños or do it in a processor; you can actually get burned by the fiery capsaicin in the peppers.

4 CUPS CHERRY TOMATOES, CUT INTO QUARTERS

1 RED BELL PEPPER, SEEDED AND CHOPPED

1 GREEN BELL PEPPER, SEEDED AND CHOPPED

½ JALAPEÑO PEPPER, SEEDED AND MINCED

½ RED ONION, CHOPPED FINE

¼ CUP CHOPPED FRESH CILANTRO LEAVES

1 TEASPOON MINCED GARLIC

½ TEASPOON GROUND CORIANDER

¼ TEASPOON GROUND CUMIN

FRESH JUICE AND ZEST OF 1 LIME

1 (15-OUNCE) CAN SODIUM-FREE BLACK BEANS,
    DRAINED AND RINSED

1. In a large bowl, thoroughly combine all the ingredients except the black beans. Add the black beans and stir to combine.

2. Serve in a bowl alongside multigrain tortillas or baked chips, or spoon over your favorite proteins, veggies, or grains.

Almond Quinoa Squares

MAKES 24 SQUARES

- ANY SEASON
- QUICK & EASY
- HIGH PROTEIN
- SUPER FOOD

This is the Clean Eating version of Rice Krispies treats, but with more flavor! You can use honey instead of brown rice syrup if you want, but use a little less, because honey is sweeter. Although brown rice syrup is high in calories, it's usually organic and is probably the best substitute for sugar if you want a sweet taste.

EXTRA-VIRGIN OLIVE OIL FOR THE BAKING DISH

1 CUP ALMOND OR CASHEW BUTTER, AT ROOM TEMPERATURE

½ CUP BROWN RICE SYRUP

2 TEASPOONS VANILLA EXTRACT

¾ CUP UNSWEETENED COCOA POWDER

12 CUPS PUFFED QUINOA

1. Lightly oil a 9-by-13-inch glass baking dish.

2. In a large bowl, stir together the almond butter, brown rice syrup, vanilla, and cocoa powder until very smooth. Stir in the puffed quinoa until it's well combined.

3. Press the mixture firmly into the baking dish and put it in the refrigerator until it's firm, about 2 hours.

4. Cut into 2-by-2-inch squares. Store in an airtight container.

Traditional Hummus

MAKES 2 CUPS

- ANY SEASON
- QUICK & EASY
- HIGH PROTEIN
- SUPER FOOD

Hummus, an ancient Middle Eastern dish, is nutrition-rich and versatile. It's a great spread and a perfect dip, and is wonderful for an energy-packed breakfast. Chickpeas (aka garbanzo beans), the main ingredient, are high in protein and free of saturated fat and cholesterol. They're also heart-friendly and help stabilize blood sugar.

3 CLOVES GARLIC

2 CUPS CANNED CHICKPEAS, DRAINED AND RINSED

½ CUP TAHINI (SESAME BUTTER)

1 TEASPOON GROUND CUMIN

1 TEASPOON GROUND CORIANDER

PINCH OF SEA SALT

FRESH JUICE AND ZEST OF 1 LEMON

1 TABLESPOON EXTRA-VIRGIN OLIVE OIL

1. Put all the ingredients into a food processor or blender and pulse until blended but not entirely smooth. Adjust the seasoning if needed.

2. Serve in a bowl as a dip for raw or steamed veggies, or use as a spread in Clean Eating sandwiches.

Oatmeal Raisin Cookies

MAKES 32 COOKIES

- ANY SEASON
- QUICK & EASY
- HIGH PROTEIN
- SUPER-FOOD

These treats are pretty close to the cookies you might find at your grandmother's house. Chewy and slightly sweet, they're perfect dunked in a glass of nonfat milk. Make sure to buy unsweetened coconut so your cookies don't turn out too sweet. These cookies freeze well, so make a double batch and just take a cookie out of the freezer when you want one.

EXTRA-VIRGIN OLIVE OIL FOR THE BAKING SHEETS
3 CUPS ROLLED OATS
1 CUP ALMOND FLOUR OR WHOLE-WHEAT FLOUR
½ CUP ALMOND BUTTER
⅓ CUP MAPLE SYRUP
1 TABLESPOON CANOLA OIL
1 TABLESPOON VANILLA
1½ CUPS UNSWEETENED APPLE JUICE
1 CUP GOLDEN RAISINS
½ CUP UNSWEETENED FLAKED OR SHREDDED COCONUT

1. Preheat the oven to 375°F.

2. Lightly coat two baking sheets with olive oil.

3. In a small bowl, combine the oats and almond flour.

4. In a large bowl, combine the almond butter, maple syrup, canola oil, vanilla, and apple juice until very well blended.

5. Add the oat mixture to the wet ingredients and stir to combine. Stir in the raisins and coconut.

6. Drop the batter by tablespoons on the baking sheets about 2 inches apart and flatten the cookies with the back of a wet spoon.

7. Bake the cookies until lightly browned, about 30 minutes. Store in an airtight container.

Clean Eating Date Bars

MAKES ABOUT 60 BARS

- ANY SEASON
- QUICK & EASY
- SUPER FOOD

Dates are extremely rich in minerals, vitamins, and fiber. They promote good digestion, help maintain bone health, counteract anemia, and provide tons of energy. Dates are also beneficial to the cardiovascular system, which makes these treats a perfect sweet choice before sports. Eating just one date a day can make a real difference in your Clean Eating plan.

EXTRA-VIRGIN OLIVE OIL FOR THE BAKING SHEET
3 CUPS PACKED PITTED DATES
¼ CUP MAPLE SYRUP
½ CUP TAHINI (SESAME BUTTER)
2 CUPS GLUTEN-FREE ROLLED OATS
⅓ CUP PECAN PIECES
1 CUP SESAME SEEDS

1. Preheat the oven to 300°F.

2. Lightly oil a rimmed baking sheet. Put the dates and maple syrup in a food processor or blender and pulse until a smooth paste forms.

3. Scrape the date mixture into a large bowl and add the tahini, oats, and pecan pieces. Stir the ingredients together thoroughly and press the mixture onto the baking sheet. Scatter the sesame seeds over the top and press them in firmly.

4. Put the baking sheet in the refrigerator until the bars are firm, about 2 hours.

5. Cut into 1-by-3-inch bars. Store the squares in the fridge or freezer in airtight containers.

Pumpkin Protein Bars

MAKES 16 BARS

- ANY SEASON
- QUICK & EASY
- BUDGET-FRIENDLY
- HIGH PROTEIN
- SUPER FOOD

Commercially prepared protein bars are often the snack of choice for people trying to eat healthfully, but these homemade ones are much tastier. When buying the whey protein powder for this recipe, look for a product from hormone-, antibiotic-, and steroid-free milk whey, or find a high-quality vegetable whey. If you don't like vanilla, you can use unflavored or chocolate protein powder with delicious results.

EXTRA-VIRGIN OLIVE OIL FOR THE BAKING DISH

1½ CUPS ROLLED OATS

1 CUP VANILLA WHEY POWDER

1 TEASPOON GROUND CINNAMON

½ TEASPOON GROUND NUTMEG

¼ TEASPOON GROUND CLOVES

¼ TEASPOON GROUND GINGER

1 CUP ALMOND BUTTER

½ CUP CANNED UNSWEETENED PUMPKIN (NOT PUMPKIN PIE MIX)

½ CUP MAPLE SYRUP

⅓ CUP UNSWEETENED APPLE SAUCE

1. Preheat the oven to 350°F.

2. Lightly oil a 9-by-13-inch baking dish or line it with parchment paper.

continued ▶

3. In a medium bowl, stir together the oats, whey powder, and spices until well combined.

4. In a small bowl, stir together the almond butter, pumpkin, maple syrup, and applesauce until blended. Pour the wet ingredients into the dry ingredients and mix well.

5. Spread the dough evenly in the baking dish so that it's about ½-inch deep.

6. Bake for about 20 minutes, or until golden brown.

7. Remove the dish from the oven and allow the slab to cool for 15 minutes before cutting it into bars. Allow to the bars to cool completely and store them in an airtight container.

Kiwi Cucumber Salsa

MAKES 3 CUPS

- WINTER/SPRING
- QUICK & EASY
- BUDGET-FRIENDLY
- LOW-FAT
- SUPER FOOD

Several shades of green make this salsa simply gorgeous, and its fresh, tart flavor is nice on baked pita bread or fish. Kiwi is incredibly high in fiber (it has more than bran), has no fat, and has a low glycemic index. It can give you an energy boost while helping to lower your blood pressure and bad cholesterol level. This salsa would be a wonderful midmorning pick-me-up during a hectic day.

4 KIWIS, PEELED AND DICED
½ ENGLISH CUCUMBER, DICED
½ RED BELL PEPPER, DICED
1 TOMATO, SEEDED AND DICED
1 TABLESPOON CHOPPED FRESH CILANTRO
¼ TEASPOON CHOPPED JALAPEÑO PEPPER
FRESH JUICE AND ZEST OF 1 LIME
PINCH OF SEA SALT

1. In a medium bowl, combine all the ingredients.

2. Store the salsa in the fridge until you're ready to eat it.

3. Serve with raw or steamed veggies or baked tortilla chips, or spoon it over your favorite protein.

Mango Pineapple Ice Pops

MAKES 8 POPS

- SPRING/SUMMER
- QUICK & EASY
- BUDGET-FRIENDLY
- LOW-FAT
- SUPER FOOD

Mango has a distinct sweet, piney taste that blends sublimely with the slightly tart flavor of pineapple. Packed with nutritional benefits, mangoes support heart health, reduce the risk of cancer, improve the digestive system, stabilize blood sugar, and boost the immune system. No wonder mango is called the "king of fruits"! If you don't have ice pop molds, you can make the pops in plastic cups (buy the sticks at your craft store).

2 POUNDS MANGO CHUNKS
1 CUP PINEAPPLE JUICE
1 CUP FRESHLY SQUEEZED ORANGE JUICE
¼ CUP FRESHLY SQUEEZED LIME JUICE

1. Put all the ingredients in a blender and puree until smooth.

2. Pour the mixture into ice pop molds or plastic cups and freeze for 4 to 6 hours. Unmold the pops by briefly running warm water on the sides of the molds or cups. Eat immediately.

Papaya Coconut Chia Pudding

SERVES 4

- ANY SEASON
- QUICK & EASY
- SUPER FOOD

Papaya was described by Christopher Columbus as the food of angels, and no wonder: its vibrant orange flesh has a smooth, buttery texture. It's also fantastic for your digestion. Don't buy green, unripe papayas because they will never ripen enough at home to be perfect. Instead, choose fruit that gives a little when squeezed, and ripen it a little further for a couple of days at room temperature.

1 CUP UNSWEETENED ALMOND MILK

1 CUP SEEDED, PEELED, AND DICED FRESH PAPAYA

2 TABLESPOONS CHIA SEEDS

2 TABLESPOONS UNSWEETENED SHREDDED COCONUT

3 TEASPOONS HONEY

1. In a medium bowl, mix together all the ingredients until well combined.

2. Cover the bowl and refrigerate for at least 6 hours, or overnight. Spoon the pudding into bowls and serve chilled.

Chocolate Protein Bites

MAKES 24 BITES

- ANY SEASON
- QUICK & EASY
- HIGH PROTEIN
- SUPER FOOD

These are like Clean Eating truffles. The base is oats, which obviously aren't in real chocolate truffles, but they add texture and nutrition to these treats. Because oats are hulled but still retain their bran and germ, they're a great source of fiber and nutrients. Oats help lower cholesterol, reduce the risk of cardiovascular disease, and stabilize blood sugar. They're truly a super food.

¾ CUP ALMOND BUTTER

¼ CUP BROWN RICE SYRUP

1 TEASPOON PURE VANILLA EXTRACT

1 CUP ROLLED LARGE-FLAKE OATS

½ CUP UNSWEETENED SHREDDED COCONUT

½ CUP CHOCOLATE PROTEIN POWDER

½ CUP DRIED CRANBERRIES

¼ CUP UNSWEETENED COCOA POWDER

PINCH OF SEA SALT

1. In a small saucepan over low heat, stir together the almond butter and brown rice syrup until melted.

2. Remove the mixture from the heat and stir in the vanilla.

3. In a large bowl, stir together the oats, coconut, protein powder, cranberries, cocoa, and salt until well combined.

4. Add the almond butter mixture to the oat mixture and combine thoroughly.

5. Put the bowl in the refrigerator and chill the paste for about 1 hour, or until you can easily roll it between your palms without it falling apart.

6. Roll into 1½-inch balls. Store the bites in an airtight container in the fridge.

Cantaloupe Ice Cream

MAKES 4 CUPS

- SUMMER
- QUICK & EASY
- BUDGET-FRIENDLY
- SUPER FOOD

This ice cream is pastel orange and subtly sweet. Cantaloupes are very high in vitamin A, vitamin C, and beta-carotene. In order to get a nice ripe melon, make sure you buy one with no gray or green shades on the skin.

3 CUPS COCONUT OR ALMOND MILK
½ CANTALOUPE, PEELED, SEEDED, AND DICED
¼ CUP HONEY

1. Pulse all the ingredients in a food processor or blender until very smooth.

2. Pour the mixture into an ice cream maker and freeze according to the manufacturer's instructions.

3. Store the ice cream in an airtight container in the freezer until you're ready to eat it.

4. Scoop into bowls and serve immediately.

Clean Berry Parfait

SERVES 4

- SUMMER
- BUDGET-FRIENDLY
- HIGH PROTEIN
- SUPER FOOD

This simple snack is an absolute treat, especially midmorning—and it's guilt-free. You can use store-bought granola as long as it's Clean Eating–friendly, but since it's so easy to make granola, why not use your own?

2 CUPS NONFAT PLAIN GREEK YOGURT

2 CUPS CLEAN EATING GRANOLA (SEE THE RECIPE IN CHAPTER 7)

4 CUPS MIXED BERRIES OF YOUR CHOICE

1. Spoon the ingredients into 4 glasses in alternating layers: yogurt on the bottom, then granola, berries, yogurt, granola, berries, yogurt, and granola.

2. Chill and serve.

Orange Cream Ice Pops

MAKES 12 POPS

- ANY SEASON
- BUDGET-FRIENDLY
- SUPER FOOD

This creamy, cool treat is flavored with real oranges. The sweetness of oranges is often hard to gauge, so leave out the honey until you taste the mixture. Then add the honey a tablespoon at a time until you reach the desired sweetness. If your oranges are very ripe and juicy, you might not need any honey at all.

4 SEEDLESS ORANGES, PEELED AND SECTIONED INTO SEGMENTS
1 CUP NONFAT PLAIN GREEK YOGURT
4 TABLESPOONS ALMOND BUTTER
3 TABLESPOONS HONEY

1. Put all the ingredients in a food processor or blender and process until smooth.

2. Pour the mixture into ice pop molds or plastic cups and freeze for 6 to 8 hours. Unmold the pops by briefly running warm water on the sides of the molds or cups. Eat immediately.

CHAPTER NINE

Salads

Green Lentil Salad

SERVES 6

- SUMMER/FALL
- QUICK & EASY
- SUPER FOOD

You might be surprised by this pretty salad's faint taste of licorice, which comes from the addition of fennel. Fennel is a pale, bulbous vegetable related to dill and carrots, with lovely feathery greens. It's a great source of vitamin C and fiber, contributing to a healthy immune system and lower cholesterol levels.

FOR THE DRESSING:

⅓ CUP FRESHLY SQUEEZED LEMON JUICE

¼ CUP EXTRA-VIRGIN OLIVE OIL

1 TABLESPOON MINCED GARLIC

2 TEASPOONS DRIED OREGANO

FRESHLY GROUND BLACK PEPPER

FOR THE SALAD:

4 CUPS CANNED GREEN LENTILS, DRAINED AND RINSED

2 TOMATOES, DICED

1 RED BELL PEPPER, SEEDED AND CUT INTO VERY NARROW STRIPS

1 CUP FINELY SLICED FENNEL

½ DICED RED ONION

½ CUP QUARTERED CANNED, WATER-PACKED, DRAINED ARTICHOKE HEARTS

SEA SALT AND FRESHLY GROUND BLACK PEPPER

½ CUP CHOPPED FRESH FLAT-LEAF PARSLEY

To make the dressing:

1. In a small bowl, whisk together the lemon juice, oil, garlic, and oregano until well combined. Season with the pepper. Set aside.

To make the salad:

1. In a large bowl, toss together the lentils, tomatoes, bell pepper, fennel, onion, and artichokes. Add the dressing to the salad and mix well.

2. Season the salad with salt and black pepper and top with parsley.

3. This salad can be refrigerated for up to 3 days.

Lemon Brown Rice Salad

SERVES 3

- SUMMER
- QUICK & EASY
- BUDGET-FRIENDLY
- HIGH PROTEIN

This is a very filling salad, so you won't need a large portion to be satisfied. The combination of the brown rice and chicken breast makes it a perfect Clean Eating balance of protein and complex carbohydrates. You'll be using a lot of skinless, boneless chicken breasts when eating cleanly, so it's efficient to bake or poach several at a time and store them in the fridge until you need them.

FOR THE SALAD:

2 CUPS COOKED BROWN RICE

1 CUP CHOPPED COOKED SKINLESS, BONELESS CHICKEN BREASTS

2 GREEN ONIONS, SLICED THINLY

1 PINT CHERRY TOMATOES, HALVED

1 CUP 1-INCH PIECES GREEN BEANS

2 TABLESPOONS CHOPPED FRESH PARSLEY

FOR THE DRESSING:

2 TABLESPOONS FRESHLY SQUEEZED LEMON JUICE

1 TABLESPOON DIJON MUSTARD

½ GARLIC CLOVE, CRUSHED

2 TABLESPOONS EXTRA-VIRGIN OLIVE OIL

FRESHLY GROUND BLACK PEPPER

To make the salad:

1. In a large bowl, combine all the ingredients and stir to combine.

To make the dressing:

1. In a small bowl, whisk together all the ingredients except the pepper.

2. Add the dressing to the salad and stir to combine. Season with the pepper.

3. Serve warm or cold.

Chicken Pecan Salad

SERVES 6

- ■ SUMMER/FALL
- ■ QUICK & EASY
- ■ HIGH PROTEIN

This elegant salad uses few ingredients to create a rich, complex flavor. Arugula is a peppery green that looks a little like dandelion leaves and is called rocket in some countries. It's extremely nutritious and is a great source of iron, folic acid, and vitamin K, so include it in your diet whenever possible. Just make sure to wash it thoroughly because arugula can be quite sandy.

FOR THE DRESSING:

2 TEASPOONS GRAINY MUSTARD

2 TEASPOONS HONEY

3 TEASPOONS APPLE CIDER VINEGAR

¼ CUP EXTRA-VIRGIN OLIVE OIL

FRESHLY GROUND BLACK PEPPER

FOR THE SALAD:

5 CUPS ARUGULA

1 TOMATO, CHOPPED

½ RED ONION, SLICED THINLY

2 SKINLESS, BONELESS CHICKEN BREASTS, COOKED AND SLICED

½ CUP CHOPPED PECANS

½ CUP CRUMBLED LOW-SODIUM FETA

To make the dressing:

1. In a small bowl, whisk together all the ingredients, seasoning with the pepper.

To make the salad:

In a large bowl, toss the arugula, tomato, and red onion with half the dressing. Put the salad on a serving platter.

3. Arrange the chicken over the salad and top with the pecans and feta.

4. Drizzle the rest of the dressing over the salad and serve.

Grilled Vegetable Pasta Salad

SERVES 6

- SUMMER/FALL
- BUDGET-FRIENDLY
- SUPER FOOD

This salad is a meal, not a starter, and will involve a little more preparation. The grilled vegetables can be prepared the day before to save time. Make some extra vegetables while you're at it to set aside for tasty wraps and frittata fillings.

FOR THE DRESSING:

¼ CUP CANOLA OIL

FRESH JUICE OF 1 LEMON

2 TABLESPOONS APPLE CIDER VINEGAR

2 TABLESPOONS CHOPPED FRESH BASIL

2 TABLESPOONS CHOPPED FRESH OREGANO

1 TEASPOON DIJON MUSTARD

FRESHLY GROUND BLACK PEPPER

FOR THE SALAD:

1 TABLESPOON EXTRA-VIRGIN OLIVE OIL

1 RED ONION, SLICED

1 EGGPLANT, CUT INTO 1-INCH SLICES

1 RED BELL PEPPER, CUT IN HALF AND SEEDED

1 ORANGE BELL PEPPER, CUT IN HALF AND SEEDED

1 GREEN ZUCCHINI, SLICED LENGTHWISE INTO ½-INCH SLABS

1 YELLOW SUMMER SQUASH, SLICED LENGTHWISE INTO ½-INCH SLABS

2 CUPS BLANCHED, HALVED GREEN BEANS

2 CUPS HALVED CHERRY TOMATOES

1 (12-OUNCE) PACKAGE WHOLE-WHEAT PENNE, COOKED
    PER PACKAGE DIRECTIONS

¼ CUP CRUMBLED LOW-SODIUM FETA

To make the dressing:

1. In a small bowl, whisk together the oil, lemon juice, vinegar, basil, oregano, and mustard. Season with the pepper and set aside.

To make the salad:

1. Preheat the grill to medium heat.

2. In a large bowl, combine the oil, onion, eggplant, peppers, zucchini, and yellow squash; toss to coat.

3. Grill the vegetables, turning occasionally, until crisp-tender and slightly charred, about 5 minutes.

4. Let the vegetables cool slightly and chop them coarsely.

5. In a large bowl, stir together the grilled vegetables, green beans, tomatoes, and pasta. Add the dressing and toss to combine. Transfer to a serving platter and top with feta.

6. Refrigerate until chilled, then serve.

Watermelon and Mint Salad

SERVES 6

- ■ SUMMER
- ■ QUICK & EASY
- ■ BUDGET-FRIENDLY
- ■ SUPER FOOD

With its pastel colors and varied textures, this is one of the loveliest salads that will ever grace your plate. The mint adds just the right freshness and zip to the flavor. Mint is often used to help promote a healthy digestive system, alleviate headaches, and combat fatigue. Buy fresh mint leaves with no brown spots or edges, and no hint of limpness.

FOR THE DRESSING:
1 TABLESPOON RED WINE VINEGAR
1 TABLESPOON EXTRA-VIRGIN OLIVE OIL
PINCH OF FRESHLY GROUND BLACK PEPPER

FOR THE SALAD:
⅓ SEEDLESS WATERMELON, RIND CUT OFF AND FLESH CUT INTO CUBES
2 CUPS HALVED CHERRY TOMATOES
4 CELERY STALKS, SLICED
½ FENNEL BULB, SHAVED OR SLICED VERY THIN
½ RED ONION, SLICED THIN
1 BUNCH MINT, CHOPPED

To make the dressing:

1. In a small bowl, whisk together the vinegar and oil. Season with the pepper and set aside.

To make the salad:

1. In a large bowl, combine all the ingredients.

2. Add the dressing to the salad and toss to mix well.

3. Chill completely and serve.

Moroccan-Style Carrot Salad

SERVES 4

- SUMMER/FALL
- BUDGET-FRIENDLY
- SUPER FOOD

Although you probably think of carrots as bright orange, they actually can be white, yellow, red, or purple. If you can find different-colored carrots, they will make a nice multihued variation of this tasty salad. The high beta-carotene content of carrots, which is responsible for their bright colors, helps cut your risk of cardiovascular disease quite significantly, even if you eat as little as a quarter cup of sliced carrots a day.

15 CARROTS, CUT INTO DISKS

2 TABLESPOONS RICE VINEGAR

2 TABLESPOONS CHOPPED FRESH PARSLEY

1 TABLESPOON HONEY

1 TABLESPOON EXTRA-VIRGIN OLIVE OIL

1 TABLESPOON MINCED GARLIC

3 TEASPOONS CHOPPED FRESH CILANTRO

1 TEASPOON GROUND CUMIN

1 TEASPOON GROUND CORIANDER

1 TEASPOON DIJON MUSTARD

FRESHLY GROUND BLACK PEPPER

⅓ CUP GOLDEN RAISINS

⅓ CUP CHOPPED ALMONDS

1. Bring a large pot of water to a boil over high heat. Add the carrots and cook until al dente, about 5 minutes.

2. Drain the hot water and run cold water into the pot until the carrots are chilled. Drain and transfer the carrots to a large bowl.

continued ▶

3. In a small bowl, whisk together all the other ingredients except the raisins and almonds.

4. Pour the dressing over the carrots and toss to coat. Add the raisins and almonds and stir to combine.

5. Allow the salad to sit for at least 4 hours in the fridge before serving to allow the spices to infuse.

Roasted Corn and Black Bean Salad

SERVES 4

- SUMMER/FALL
- BUDGET-FRIENDLY
- LOW-FAT
- SUPER FOOD

Corn on the cob is at its finest when grilled, though people more often steam or blanch it in hot water. Grilling brings out the sweetness of the corn and adds a pleasing charred taste that's perfect for this colorful salad. The key to good flavor is to cook the corn while it's as fresh as possible, preferably on the day it's picked or at least within a few days. Avoid ears with dry-looking or wilted husks.

4 CORN COBS, HUSK ON AND SOAKED IN WATER FOR AT LEAST 2 HOURS

2 (15-OUNCE) CANS SODIUM-FREE BLACK BEANS, DRAINED AND RINSED

1 RED BELL PEPPER, SEEDED AND DICED

1 GREEN PEPPER, SEEDED AND DICED

1 RED ONION, DICED

½ ENGLISH CUCUMBER, DICED

1 JALAPEÑO PEPPER, SEEDED AND FINELY CHOPPED

4 TABLESPOONS CHOPPED CILANTRO

FRESH JUICE OF 2 LIMES

1 TEASPOON GROUND CUMIN

1. Preheat the grill to medium heat.

2. Put the soaked corn over the fire and grill it until the husks are blackened and the kernels are very tender.

3. Remove the cobs from the grill and allow them to cool.

4. Shuck the corn and use a sharp knife to shave off the kernels into large bowl. Add the rest of the ingredients and toss to combine.

5. Chill completely in the fridge and serve.

Moroccan Lentil Salad

SERVES 6

- SUMMER
- QUICK & EASY
- HIGH PROTEIN
- SUPER FOOD

This perfect picnic salad takes little time to prepare and will give you energy to chase Frisbees, swim, or hike all afternoon. There are many wonderful canned lentils on the market that contain no sodium or additives and are easy to use in this recipe. Simply read the labels to find the brand that works for you. If you don't like canned lentils, you can cook your own from the dry form.

2 (15-OUNCE) CANS SODIUM-FREE LENTILS, DRAINED AND RINSED

1 (15-OUNCE) CAN SODIUM-FREE CHICKPEAS, DRAINED AND RINSED

1 RED BELL PEPPER, SEEDED AND CHOPPED

1 YELLOW BELL PEPPER, SEEDED AND CHOPPED

2 TOMATOES, SEEDED AND CHOPPED

½ CUCUMBER, CHOPPED

3 GREEN ONIONS, CHOPPED

1 JALAPEÑO PEPPER, MINCED

FRESH JUICE OF 2 LIMES

1 TEASPOON GROUND CUMIN

½ TEASPOON ALLSPICE

¼ CUP CHOPPED FRESH CILANTRO

1. Combine all the ingredients in a large bowl and stir to combine.

2. Chill the salad for at least 30 minutes before serving.

Peach Beet Salad

SERVES 4

- ■ SUMMER/FALL/WINTER
- ■ LOW-FAT
- ■ SUPER FOOD

Lots of people love beets, but you might not if you've never tasted them roasted or steamed very gently. These vibrant, earthy root vegetables can be messy to prepare, because when you peel them, they tend to stain everything they touch. But it's entirely worth the trouble. When you buy your beets, try to get them with their greens still attached; you can cut those off and use them in a tasty salad or braised as a side dish.

2 BEETS

4 CUPS ARUGULA

1 TABLESPOON CHOPPED FRESH BASIL

1 TEASPOON CHOPPED FRESH THYME

1 TABLESPOON SHERRY VINEGAR

1 TABLESPOON EXTRA-VIRGIN OLIVE OIL

1 TEASPOON HONEY

FRESHLY GROUND BLACK PEPPER

2 PEACHES, PITTED AND CUT INTO THIN WEDGES

1. Preheat the oven to 350°F.

2. Fill a baking dish with about 1/2 inch of water.

3. Put the beets in the dish, cover, and bake for about 60 minutes, until the beets are tender.

4. Remove the beets from the dish and allow them to cool most of the way.

5. Peel off the skins with a sharp knife and dice the beets.

continued ▶

Peach Beet Salad *continued* ▶

6. In a large bowl, toss together the arugula, basil, and thyme.

7. In a small bowl, whisk together the vinegar, oil, and honey until well combined. Season with the pepper. Add the dressing to the greens and toss to combine.

8. Divide the greens among 4 plates. Top with the beets and peaches and serve.

Mushroom Beet Green Salad

SERVES 4

- FALL/WINTER
- BUDGET-FRIENDLY
- HIGH PROTEIN
- SUPER FOOD

This salad is the perfect dish if you suspect a cold is coming on or if you just feel under the weather. Every element boosts your immunity, and the combination of ingredients includes almost every vitamin, including a double dose of vitamin C. You can use asiago cheese instead of reduced-sodium feta, if you prefer.

4 CUPS BABY SPINACH LEAVES

2 CUPS SLICED BUTTON MUSHROOMS

1 SEEDLESS ORANGE, PEELED, SEGMENTED, AND CHOPPED

FRESH JUICE AND ZEST OF 1 LEMON

1 TABLESPOON EXTRA-VIRGIN OLIVE OIL

FRESHLY GROUND BLACK PEPPER

1 TABLESPOON CRUMBLED LOW-SODIUM FETA

1. In a large bowl, toss together the spinach, mushrooms, and orange.

2. In a small bowl, whisk together the lemon juice, zest, and oil. Season with the pepper.

3. Toss the dressing with the greens and divide the salad among 4 plates. Top with feta and serve.

CHAPTER TEN

Vegetables

Slow Cooker Sweet Potatoes

SERVES 8

- FALL/WINTER
- QUICK & EASY
- LOW-FAT
- SUPER FOOD

Although you might think of sweet potatoes as orange in color, they can also be white, purple, or yellow. Any sweet potato color will work well in this delicious side dish; combine them for an extra-festive result. Sweet potatoes contain more than 400 percent of the RDA of vitamin A and are packed with antioxidants. You might be inclined to avoid this starchy vegetable, but sweet potatoes are quite healthful for people with diabetes and can actually improve blood sugar levels.

8 SWEET POTATOES, PEELED AND DICED INTO LARGE CHUNKS
½ CUP UNSWEETENED APPLE JUICE
2 TABLESPOONS MAPLE SYRUP
½ TEASPOON ALLSPICE
½ TEASPOON GROUND GINGER
¼ TEASPOON GROUND CINNAMON
¼ TEASPOON GROUND NUTMEG
FRESHLY GROUND BLACK PEPPER

1. Turn a slow cooker on low heat.

2. In a large bowl, combine all the ingredients except the pepper and mix well.

3. Put mixture in the slow cooker. Cover the slow cooker and cook on low heat for 7 to 8 hours, until tender.

4. Put the potatoes in a bowl and season with the pepper. Serve alongside chicken or pork.

Garlic Green Beans

SERVES 6

- SUMMER
- QUICK & EASY
- LOW-SODIUM
- BUDGET-FRIENDLY

There's a lot of garlic in this dish, but when you cook it on low heat until it's softened and almost caramelized, garlic becomes deliciously sweet. Garlic is a health superstar with powerful anticancer properties, and it's used to treat bacterial infections. A head of garlic can keep for up to a month if stored in a cool, dark place in a loosely covered container.

1 TABLESPOON EXTRA-VIRGIN OLIVE OIL
2 TABLESPOONS MINCED GARLIC
3 POUNDS FRESH GREEN BEANS
FRESHLY GROUND BLACK PEPPER

1. Put the oil in a large skillet over medium heat.

2. Add the garlic and cook until fragrant, golden brown, and almost roasted, about 4 minutes. Set aside.

3. Bring a large pot of water to a boil. Add the beans, cover the pot, and cook until crisp-tender, 8 to 10 minutes.

4. Drain the beans and put them in the skillet with the garlic. Toss to coat, season with the pepper, and heat the veggies over medium heat.

5. Serve hot, alongside your favorite protein.

Edamame Succotash

SERVES 6

- SUMMER
- HIGH PROTEIN
- LOW-SODIUM
- SUPER FOOD

Succotash usually contains lima beans, but this variation uses edamame instead. Edamame—soy beans that are still in the pod—are usually served as a finger food on their own, steamed and salted in their shells. They're a complete protein and are very high in antioxidants and fiber. This means that edamame improves the immune system, helps prevent certain cancers, boosts the metabolism, and can help prevent food cravings.

1 TEASPOON EXTRA-VIRGIN OLIVE OIL

1 RED BELL PEPPER, SEEDED AND DICED

¼ SWEET ONION, CHOPPED

2 TEASPOONS MINCED GARLIC

2 TABLESPOONS WATER

2 CUPS FRESH CORN KERNELS (ABOUT 4 EARS)

1 CUP FROZEN OR REFRIGERATED SHELLED EDAMAME,
    COOKED PER PACKAGE DIRECTIONS

3 TEASPOONS APPLE CIDER VINEGAR

2 TABLESPOONS CHOPPED FRESH PARSLEY

2 TABLESPOONS CHOPPED FRESH BASIL

FRESHLY GROUND BLACK PEPPER

1. Place a large skillet over medium heat and add the oil.

2. Sauté the bell pepper, onion, and garlic until the vegetables are softened, about 5 minutes.

continued ▶

3. Add the water, corn, and edamame and cook for about 5 minutes, stirring occasionally.

4. Remove the vegetables from the heat and stir in the vinegar, parsley, and basil. Season with the pepper.

5. Serve warm alongside fish, chicken, or pork.

Brussels Sprouts with Lemon

- ■ AUTUMN/WINTER
- ■ QUICK & EASY
- ■ LOW-SODIUM
- ■ BUDGET-FRIENDLY
- ■ SUPER FOOD

Brussels sprouts belong high on the Clean Eating food list. They're packed with protein, although it's incomplete protein—if you combine Brussels sprouts with whole grains, the result is a complete protein that provides all the amino acids your body needs. Brussels sprouts are also a great source of fiber, vitamin A, folate, calcium, and potassium.

½ CUP WATER
5 CUPS QUARTERED BRUSSELS SPROUTS
SEA SALT AND FRESHLY GROUND BLACK PEPPER
1 TABLESPOON EXTRA-VIRGIN OLIVE OIL
1 TABLESPOON FRESHLY SQUEEZED LEMON JUICE
1 TEASPOON LEMON ZEST

1. Put the water and Brussels sprouts in a large skillet over medium heat. Bring to a simmer and cover the skillet.

2. Cook until the Brussels sprouts are tender but still crisp, 5 to 8 minutes. Most of the water should be evaporated. Season with a pinch of the salt and pepper.

3. Increase the heat to medium-high and add the oil to the skillet.

4. Cook without stirring for about 5 minutes, until the Brussels sprouts are lightly caramelized on the underside.

5. Remove the skillet from the heat and stir in the lemon juice and zest. Serve alongside chicken or beef.

Pumpkin with Sage

SERVES 6

- **FALL/WINTER**
- **BUDGET-FRIENDLY**
- **SUPER FOOD**

Many people use pumpkin only for breads and pies, but it's also a lovely side dish or main course. Keep in mind that you don't want to cook the field pumpkins that you buy from a big farm stand or supermarket for carving into Halloween jack-o'-lanterns. Ask your produce seller for good cooking varieties. You can store uncut cooking pumpkins in a cool, dry spot for up to two months.

2 TABLESPOONS EXTRA-VIRGIN OLIVE OIL, PLUS MORE
    FOR THE BAKING SHEET
1 (4-POUND) COOKING PUMPKIN, PEELED, SEEDED, AND
    CUT INTO 1½-INCH CHUNKS
2 TEASPOONS CHOPPED FRESH SAGE LEAVES
SEA SALT AND FRESHLY GROUND BLACK PEPPER

1. Preheat the oven to 450°F.

2. Oil a baking sheet or line it with parchment paper.

3. In a large bowl, toss the pumpkin, 2 tablespoons oil, and sage until well combined.

4. Put the pumpkin mixture on the baking sheet and lightly season with salt and pepper.

5. Bake, stirring once, until the pumpkin is tender and lightly caramelized, about 30 minutes. Serve alongside chicken or pork.

Swiss Chard with Garlic

SERVES 6

- SUMMER/AUTUMN
- QUICK & EASY
- LOW-SODIUM
- BUDGET-FRIENDLY
- SUPER FOOD

Swiss chard isn't as popular as its dark leafy counterpart, spinach, but it ranks pretty close in nutritional value. Swiss chard contains thirteen different anti- oxidants, more than 700 percent of the RDA of vitamin K, and more than 200 percent of the RDA of vitamin A. If you buy Swiss chard with colored rather than white stems, discard the stems, because they can be very tough.

1 TABLESPOON EXTRA-VIRGIN OLIVE OIL

3 GARLIC CLOVES, THINLY SLICED

8 CUPS CHOPPED SWISS CHARD STEMS

12 CUPS ROUGHLY CHOPPED SWISS CHARD LEAVES

1 TABLESPOON HONEY

1 TABLESPOON APPLE CIDER VINEGAR

FRESHLY GROUND BLACK PEPPER

1. Place a Dutch oven or heavy saucepan over medium heat and add the oil and garlic. Sauté until fragrant, 1 to 2 minutes.

2. Stir in the stems and cook for about 5 minutes, stirring occasionally, until softened. Add the leaves and cook, covered, until the leaves are wilted, about 4 minutes.

3. Uncover and cook until all the vegetable liquid has evaporated, about 3 minutes. Stir in the honey and vinegar.

4. Season with the pepper. Serve alongside fish or beef.

Celery Root Puree

- FALL/WINTER
- QUICK & EASY
- LOW-FAT
- BUDGET-FRIENDLY

Celery root, or celeriac, tastes like celery, but in its raw state looks like a lumpy, hairy root ball. It's often crusted with dirt around its roots, so thoroughly wash and scrub it before you cut it. Celeriac is high in fiber and low in cholesterol and saturated fat. It's also a great source of riboflavin, calcium, vitamin B_6, magnesium, phosphorus, potassium, and vitamins A, C, and K.

1 CELERY ROOT, PEELED AND CUT INTO 1-INCH PIECES
2 WHITE POTATOES, PEELED AND CUT INTO 1-INCH PIECES
½ CUP COCONUT MILK
½ TEASPOON NUTMEG
PINCH OF SEA SALT

1. In a large saucepan, put the celery root and potatoes in enough cold water to cover. Bring the water to a boil over medium-high heat, then reduce the heat to a simmer.

2. Cook the vegetables until tender, 15 to 20 minutes.

3. Put the cooked vegetables, coconut milk, and nutmeg in a food processor or blender, and pulse until very smooth.

4. Season with the sea salt and serve alongside chicken or pork.

Eggplant Parmesan Bites

SERVES 4 TO 6

- SUMMER
- BUDGET-FRIENDLY
- SUPER FOOD

This rich casserole takes a bit of preparation, but it can be made ahead of time and popped into the oven when you want to eat it. Eggplant is often used as a substitute for meat because of its firm, fleshy texture. This method maximizes the effect by soaking up just a little bit of olive oil. You can eat this dish as a main course or a side dish. Eggplant is very good for brain and cardiovascular functioning.

2 EGG WHITES, BEATEN

1 CUP WHOLE-WHEAT BREADCRUMBS

1 TABLESPOON DRIED BASIL

½ TEASPOON DRIED OREGANO

1 EGGPLANT, CUT INTO ½-INCH SLICES

EXTRA-VIRGIN OLIVE OIL FOR DRIZZLING

2 TOMATOES, CHOPPED

2 TABLESPOONS FRESHLY GRATED PARMESAN

1 TABLESPOON CHOPPED PARSLEY, FOR GARNISH

1. Preheat the oven to 400°F.

2. Place a piece of parchment paper or foil on a baking sheet and set aside.

3. In a shallow bowl, add the egg whites.

4. In another shallow bowl, combine the breadcrumbs, basil, and oregano.

5. Dip each slice of eggplant into the egg whites, then dredge it in the bread-crumbs, coating both sides. Put the dredged eggplant on the baking sheet. Lightly drizzle with the oil.

continued ▶

6. Bake for about 5 minutes per side, until lightly golden.

7. Remove the eggplant from the oven and lower the heat to 350°F.

8. Put 4 of the eggplant slices on the bottom of an 8-inch-square baking dish. Sprinkle half of the tomato over the eggplant and lay the remaining eggplant slices over the tomato. Top the second eggplant layer with the remaining tomato, and sprinkle with the Parmesan.

9. Bake for 20 minutes. Serve garnished with parsley.

Sautéed Spinach

- SPRING/SUMMER/FALL
- QUICK & EASY
- BUDGET-FRIENDLY
- LOW-SODIUM
- SUPER FOOD

This dish is very simple, but it's elevated by the addition of nutmeg. The best way to add this warm spice is to grate it fresh off a nutmeg seed. Note that, unlike other spices, nutmeg should not be stored in the freezer. It also loses potency and freshness when exposed to moisture, heat, or direct sunlight.

1 TABLESPOON EXTRA-VIRGIN OLIVE OIL

4 TEASPOONS MINCED GARLIC

8 CUPS FRESH SPINACH

¼ TEASPOON NUTMEG

1. Place a large skillet over medium-high heat and add the olive oil.

2. Sauté the garlic until it's fragrant, about 2 minutes.

3. Add the spinach and cook until it's wilted, about 2 minutes.

4. Season with the nutmeg and serve alongside your favorite protein.

Balsamic Roasted Tomatoes

MAKES 6 CUPS

- ■ SUMMER
- ■ BUDGET-FRIENDLY
- ■ SUPER FOOD

Jarred sun-dried tomatoes can be expensive, so making your own version in the oven is cheaper and a great way to preserve the goodness of ripe tomatoes. You don't have to use balsamic vinegar, but it adds a rich, tangy sweetness that's sublime.

1 TABLESPOON EXTRA-VIRGIN OLIVE OIL, PLUS MORE FOR THE BAKING SHEET
16 PLUM TOMATOES, CUT INTO WEDGES
1 TABLESPOON BALSAMIC VINEGAR
1 TEASPOON DRIED BASIL
¼ TEASPOON FRESHLY GROUND BLACK PEPPER
PINCH OF SEA SALT

1. Preheat the oven to 200°F.

2. Lightly coat a baking sheet with oil and set aside.

3. Toss the tomatoes, 1 tablespoon oil, vinegar, basil, pepper, and salt in a large bowl until well coated. Arrange the tomatoes, cut side up, on the baking sheet.

4. Roast until tender and chewy, about 8 hours or overnight.

5. Use the roasted tomatoes in just about any recipe to add zing and sweetness, or just munch on them as a snack.

Mushroom Kebabs

SERVES 4

- ANY SEASON
- QUICK & EASY
- BUDGET-FRIENDLY
- LOW-SODIUM

Portobello mushrooms have a meaty texture and rich, earthy flavor. They're also very large, which makes them ideal for barbecuing. High in fiber and low in fat, they offer a good balance between protein and carbs. Very low in calories, portobellos are perfect for Clean Eating dishes.

1 TABLESPOON BALSAMIC VINEGAR

1 TABLESPOON EXTRA-VIRGIN OLIVE OIL

1 TEASPOON FRESH CHOPPED OREGANO

4 PORTOBELLO MUSHROOMS, QUARTERED

4 WOODEN SKEWERS, SOAKED IN WATER FOR 30 MINUTES

1. In a medium bowl, whisk together the vinegar, oil, and oregano. Add the mushrooms and toss to coat. Marinate in the fridge for at least 60 minutes.

2. Preheat the grill to medium-high.

3. Thread the marinated mushrooms onto the skewers. Grill the mushrooms 5 minutes per side, turning once.

4. Serve alongside beef.

Spicy Grilled Corn on the Cob

SERVES 6

- SUMMER/FALL
- QUICK & EASY
- BUDGET-FRIENDLY
- LOW-SODIUM
- SUPER FOOD

Cayenne pepper gives this corn a nice, hot kick. This spice has been around for more than seven thousand years and has been used for medicinal as well as culinary purposes. Cayenne can actually be a valuable part of a weight-loss plan because it increases your metabolism for as much as twenty minutes after you eat it, helping to burn fat. It's also heart-friendly and can boost the immune system.

6 SHUCKED FRESH CORN COBS, WITH THE STEM INTACT
2 TEASPOONS UNSALTED BUTTER
FRESH JUICE AND ZEST OF 1 LIME
½ TEASPOON CAYENNE PEPPER

1. Preheat the grill to high heat.

2. Grill the corn, turning, until it chars lightly on all sides, 10 to 12 minutes.

3. Brush the corn with the butter and sprinkle evenly with the juice, zest, and cayenne pepper.

4. Serve immediately alongside your favorite protein.

New Potatoes and Asparagus

SERVES 6

- ■ SPRING
- ■ BUDGET-FRIENDLY
- ■ LOW-SODIUM
- ■ SUPER FOOD

This dish is like spring in a bowl. Tender, tiny potatoes are low in calories, high in fiber, and full of nutrients, especially in the skin. Potatoes have a long history as a healthful food, and were eaten by sailors in the eighteenth century for their vitamin C, which boosts immunity and wards off the vitamin-deficiency disease scurvy. Try to buy your potatoes loose rather than in a bag so you can make sure they're blemish-free, unbruised, and thin-skinned.

1 TABLESPOON EXTRA-VIRGIN OLIVE OIL, PLUS MORE FOR THE
    BAKING SHEET
1 BUNCH FRESH ASPARAGUS, WOODY ENDS SNAPPED OFF AND
    TENDER STALKS CUT INTO 2-INCH PIECES
1 POUND NEW POTATOES, HALVED
2 GARLIC CLOVES, SLICED THINLY
1 TEASPOON DRIED BASIL
FRESHLY GROUND BLACK PEPPER
1 TABLESPOON CHOPPED FRESH PARSLEY

1. Preheat the oven to 400°F.

2. Lightly coat a baking sheet with oil and set aside.

3. In a large bowl, toss the asparagus, potatoes, 1 tablespoon oil, garlic, and basil. Season with the pepper.

4. Roast the potatoes for 40 to 45 minutes, until tender.

5. Garnish with the parsley and serve alongside your favorite protein.

Roasted Cauliflower

SERVES 4

- SUMMER/FALL
- QUICK & EASY
- BUDGET-FRIENDLY
- LOW-SODIUM
- SUPER FOOD

If you've only ever eaten cauliflower blanched, this recipe will be a real eye-opener. Cauliflower is quite easy to overcook, and boiling it can create a mushy, flavorless mess. Roasting cauliflower, by contrast, enhances the earthy taste and keeps it tender-crisp. But if you're prone to kidney stones or gout, you'll have to control yourself around this delicious dish: cauliflower contains a substance called purine, which breaks down into uric acid in the body.

1 HEAD CAULIFLOWER, CUT INTO FLORETS
EXTRA-VIRGIN OLIVE OIL FOR DRIZZLING
1 TEASPOON FRESH CHOPPED THYME
FRESHLY GROUND BLACK PEPPER

1. Preheat the oven to 450°F.

2. Line a baking sheet with parchment paper or foil. Put the cauliflower florets on the baking sheet. Drizzle with the oil and sprinkle with the thyme and pepper.

3. Bake for 20 minutes, or until tender. Serve alongside fish, chicken, or pork.

Oven-Baked Zucchini

SERVES 8

- SUMMER/FALL
- QUICK & EASY
- BUDGET-FRIENDLY
- SUPER FOOD

Maybe you've indulged in a dish of zucchini sautéed in butter until crispy, then covered in melted Parmesan. That stuff sure is delicious, but it's truly a heart attack on a plate. This healthful version is made in the oven with very little fat. You can taste the zucchini as well as the cheese, a yummy combination that makes Clean Eating fun.

1 TABLESPOON EXTRA-VIRGIN OLIVE OIL, PLUS MORE
    FOR THE BAKING SHEET
3 ZUCCHINI, CUT INTO ½-INCH SLICES
3 YELLOW ZUCCHINI, CUT INTO ½-INCH SLICES
1 TEASPOON MINCED GARLIC
½ TEASPOON FRESHLY GROUND BLACK PEPPER
2 TABLESPOONS FRESHLY GRATED PARMESAN CHEESE

1. Preheat the oven to 350°F.

2. Lightly coat a baking sheet with oil.

3. Put the zucchini, 1 tablespoon oil, garlic, and pepper in a large bowl and toss to combine well.

3. Arrange the vegetable slices on the baking sheet and sprinkle with the Parmesan.

4. Bake for about 15 minutes, until the zucchini has softened and the Parmesan has lightly browned. Serve alongside pork or beef.

CHAPTER ELEVEN

Soups and Stews

Creamy Broccoli Soup

SERVES 6

- SUMMER/FALL
- BUDGET-FRIENDLY
- SUPER FOOD

Broccoli has been the subject of more than three hundred different scientific studies of cancer-fighting foods. This super food has unique detoxifying and anti-inflammatory properties that have great potential for future cancer-prevention therapies. In fact, eating as little as half a cup of broccoli a day could reduce your risk of developing cancer. Broccoli is also a superb source of vitamin C and vitamin K.

1 TEASPOON EXTRA-VIRGIN OLIVE OIL

1 SWEET ONION, CHOPPED

1 TEASPOON MINCED GARLIC

3 HEADS BROCCOLI, CUT INTO FLORETS

2 WHITE POTATOES, PEELED AND ROUGHLY CHOPPED

8 CUPS LOW-FAT, LOW-SODIUM VEGETABLE OR CHICKEN BROTH

½ TEASPOON GRATED NUTMEG

½ CUP NONFAT PLAIN GREEK YOGURT

FRESHLY GROUND BLACK PEPPER

1. In a large pot over medium heat, add the oil, onion, and garlic. Sauté until the onion and garlic are translucent, 3 to 4 minutes.

2. Add two-thirds of the broccoli florets, potatoes, broth, and nutmeg.

3. Over high heat, bring the soup to a boil. Reduce the heat to medium-low and simmer until the vegetables are tender, about 20 minutes.

4. Working in batches if necessary, pour the soup into a food processor or blender and puree until smooth, or puree in the pot with an immersion (handheld stick) blender. Stir in the yogurt.

5. Fill a pot two-thirds full of water and bring it to a boil over medium-high heat. Blanch the remaining one-third of the broccoli florets until al dente. Drain the florets well and add them to the soup.

6. Season with the pepper and serve piping hot.

Sunny Carrot Squash Soup

SERVES 6

- SUMMER/FALL
- BUDGET-FRIENDLY
- LOW-FAT
- SUPER FOOD

This truly happy-looking soup should bring a smile to your face when you eat it. Its vibrant color is perfectly complemented by the heat of the freshly grated ginger. Before grating the ginger, peel off the tough outer skin; afterward, wash your hands thoroughly. If you want even hotter flavor, wait to add the ginger until there are only about fifteen minutes of cooking time left.

1 SWEET ONION, CHOPPED
1 TEASPOON MINCED GARLIC
1 TEASPOON EXTRA-VIRGIN OLIVE OIL
8 CUPS LOW-SODIUM VEGETABLE STOCK
2 CARROTS, PEELED AND DICED
1 BUTTERNUT SQUASH, PEELED, SEEDED, AND DICED
3 APPLES, PEELED, CORED, AND DICED
1 TEASPOON GROUND CINNAMON
1 TEASPOON GROUND NUTMEG
1 TABLESPOON FRESH GRATED GINGER ROOT
FRESHLY GROUND BLACK PEPPER

1. In a large stock pot over medium heat, sauté the onions and garlic in the oil until they are translucent, about 5 minutes.

2. Add the stock, carrots, squash, apples, cinnamon, nutmeg, and ginger.

3. Over high heat, bring the soup to a boil, then turn the heat down to medium-low and simmer for 60 minutes, or until the vegetables are tender.

4. Working in batches, puree the soup in a blender or food processor until smooth, or puree in the pot with an immersion (handheld stick) blender.

5. Return the soup to the pot and reheat, stirring and seasoning with the pepper. Serve piping hot.

Rustic Quinoa and Bean Soup

SERVES 6

- ■ FALL
- ■ QUICK & EASY
- ■ HIGH PROTEIN
- ■ SUPER FOOD

This soup can be enjoyed at any time of the year, but it has a rib-sticking heart-iness that is especially wonderful on crisp fall days. You might think the texture of the tiny quinoa would get lost in soup, but this soup isn't cooked very long, so each ingredient retains its individuality. If you're going to freeze a batch, leave the spinach out until you reheat it so that the gorgeous green color isn't lost.

1 TEASPOON CANOLA OIL

1 SWEET ONION, CHOPPED

1 TABLESPOON MINCED GARLIC

4 CELERY STALKS, CHOPPED

1 CARROT, PEELED AND DICED

1 TEASPOON GROUND CUMIN

1 TEASPOON GROUND CORIANDER

⅓ CUP DRY QUINOA, RINSED AND PICKED OVER

6 CUPS LOW-FAT, LOW-SODIUM VEGETABLE BROTH

1 (14.5-OUNCE) CAN NO-SALT DICED TOMATOES

2 CUPS DRAINED AND RINSED SODIUM-FREE CANNED WHITE KIDNEY BEANS

2 CUPS SHREDDED BABY SPINACH

1. Heat the oil in a large saucepan over medium heat and sauté the onion, garlic, celery, and carrot for 3 minutes.

2. Add the cumin, coriander, and quinoa and cook for 2 more minutes.

continued ▶

3. Pour in the broth and tomatoes and bring to a boil.

4. Reduce the heat to medium-low and simmer until the quinoa is cooked, about 15 minutes.

5. Stir in the beans and spinach. Cook until the beans are hot and the spinach is wilted, 2 to 3 minutes.

6. Serve immediately.

Old-Fashioned Vegetable Soup

SERVES 6

- ■ SUMMER/FALL
- ■ BUDGET-FRIENDLY

This simple soup made of everyday ingredients might well have graced your grandmother's stove. The thyme, which poet Rudyard Kipling wrote "smells like dawn in paradise," is a fragrant last-minute addition, the scent of which will call people to the table without prodding.

1 TEASPOON EXTRA-VIRGIN OLIVE OIL

1 SWEET ONION, FINELY CHOPPED

1 TEASPOON MINCED GARLIC

3 CELERY STALKS WITH LEAVES, FINELY CHOPPED

2 CARROTS, PEELED AND FINELY CHOPPED

8 CUPS LOW-SODIUM VEGETABLE STOCK

1 YAM, PEELED AND DICED

1 (14.5-OUNCE) CAN NO-SALT DICED TOMATOES

2 CUPS 1-INCH GREEN BEAN PIECES

1 (15-OUNCE) CAN SODIUM-FREE WHITE NAVY BEANS, DRAINED AND RINSED

2 TABLESPOONS CHOPPED FRESH THYME

FRESHLY GROUND BLACK PEPPER

1. In a large stock pot over medium heat, heat the oil and sauté the onions, garlic, celery, and carrots for 3 to 4 minutes.

2. Add the stock, yam, and tomatoes. Bring the soup to a boil, then turn down the heat and simmer for 60 minutes, or until the vegetables are tender.

3. Add the green beans, navy beans, and thyme and simmer an additional 3 to 4 minutes.

4. Season with the black pepper and serve piping hot.

Irish Bean and Cabbage Soup

SERVES 6

- SUMMER/FALL/WINTER
- QUICK & EASY
- BUDGET-FRIENDLY
- HIGH PROTEIN
- SUPER FOOD

Pure peasant food, this soup can provide energy for even the most strenuous days. The humble cabbage is a great source of vitamins C and K, folate, and cancer-preventing antioxidants. Never buy pre-shredded or pre-cut cabbage— once it's cut, it starts to lose its vitamin C. Go for a whole head instead, choosing one that's firm, heavy, shiny, and free of blemishes or cracks.

1 TEASPOON CANOLA OIL

1 SWEET ONION, CHOPPED

1 TABLESPOON MINCED GARLIC

3 CELERY STALKS WITH THEIR LEAVES, CHOPPED

1 HEAD GREEN CABBAGE, CORED AND CHOPPED FINE

2 YUKON GOLD POTATOES, PEELED AND DICED

2 CARROTS, PEELED AND SLICED INTO DISKS

1 TEASPOON DRIED THYME

1 TEASPOON DRIED OREGANO

8 CUPS LOW-FAT, LOW-SODIUM VEGETABLE BROTH

1 (14.5-OUNCE) CAN SODIUM-FREE DICED TOMATOES

1 (15-OUNCE) CAN NO-SALT WHITE NAVY BEANS, DRAINED AND RINSED

FRESHLY GROUND BLACK PEPPER

1. In a large saucepan over medium heat, heat the oil and sauté the onions, garlic, celery, cabbage, potatoes, and carrots for about 10 minutes.

2. Stir the herbs, broth, and tomatoes into the pot and bring the soup to a boil.

3. Reduce the heat to medium-low and simmer the soup until the vegetables are tender, about 20 minutes.

4. Add the beans and simmer for 5 more minutes.

5. Season with the pepper and serve immediately.

Roasted Pepper and Lentil Soup

SERVES 8

- SUMMER/FALL
- HIGH PROTEIN
- SUPER FOOD

This isn't a soup you can whip together in half an hour, unless you roast your peppers ahead of time and store them in your fridge. Some people have an intolerance to bell peppers (which can result in minor to severe reactions) and might want to avoid this soup. But if you can eat peppers, go for it: they contain almost 200 percent of the RDA of vitamin C and are a great source of vitamin A, vitamin B_6, and folate.

6 RED BELL PEPPERS, CUT IN HALF AND SEEDED

6 YELLOW BELL PEPPERS, CUT IN HALF AND SEEDED

1 SWEET ONION, CHOPPED

3 GARLIC CLOVES, LIGHTLY CRUSHED

2 TABLESPOONS EXTRA-VIRGIN OLIVE OIL

FRESHLY GROUND BLACK PEPPER

1 (6-OUNCE) CAN LOW-SODIUM TOMATO PASTE

8 CUPS LOW-SODIUM VEGETABLE STOCK

1 CARROT, PEELED AND DICED

2 CELERY STALKS, DICED

2 CUPS LENTILS, DRAINED AND RINSED

4 TABLESPOONS LOW-FAT PLAIN GREEK YOGURT

2 TABLESPOONS CHOPPED FRESH BASIL

1. Preheat the oven to 350°F.

2. Line a large baking sheet with foil and arrange the bell peppers, onion, and garlic on it. Drizzle the vegetables with the oil and season with the black pepper. Roast for 20 minutes, or until the vegetables are soft.

3. Remove the vegetables from the oven and allow them to cool enough to be handled.

4. Puree the vegetables in a food processor or blender until smooth.

5. In a large stockpot over medium-high heat, bring the puree, tomato paste, stock, carrots, and celery to a boil.

6. Reduce the heat to medium-low and simmer the soup until the vegetables are tender, about 30 minutes.

7. Stir in the lentils and simmer an additional 5 minutes.

8. Season with the black pepper and serve topped with the yogurt and fresh basil.

Turkey Split Pea Soup

SERVES 6

- FALL/WINTER
- HIGH PROTEIN
- SUPER FOOD

Turkey isn't the first thing that comes to mind when people think of pea soup; more often it's ham or bacon. But turkey combines beautifully with the peas and the thick heartiness of this soup. When possible, use an organic, pasture-raised bird that's free of antibiotics and steroids; its meat is cleaner and more nutritious.

1 TEASPOON EXTRA-VIRGIN OLIVE OIL
1 SWEET ONION, CHOPPED
1 TEASPOON MINCED GARLIC
8 CUPS LOW-SODIUM VEGETABLE STOCK
3 CUPS DRY SPLIT PEAS, RINSED AND PICKED OVER
4 CELERY STALKS WITH THEIR LEAVES, CHOPPED
3 CARROTS, PEELED AND DICED
2 POTATOES, PEELED AND DICED
2 BAY LEAVES
2 TEASPOONS CHOPPED FRESH THYME
1 CUP DICED, LEAN TURKEY BREAST
FRESHLY GROUND BLACK PEPPER

1. In a large soup pot over medium-high heat, heat the oil and sauté the onion and garlic until translucent, about 5 minutes.

2. Add the stock and peas. Bring to a boil, then reduce the heat to medium-low.

3. Simmer for 2 hours, then add the remaining vegetables, bay leaves, and thyme.

4. Simmer another 60 minutes, or until the peas and vegetables are soft. Add the turkey and heat until it's warmed through. Remove the bay leaves.

5. Season with the pepper and serve piping hot.

Lentil and Sweet Potato Stew

SERVES 6

- FALL/WINTER
- BUDGET-FRIENDLY
- SUPER FOOD

Yams and sweet potatoes are often thought to be the same thing, but they're not—they're not even related! Yams are a dark, tough-skinned tuber from a tropical vine, while sweet potatoes, a root, have a lighter color and thinner skin. Almost anything labeled a "yam" in your supermarket is actually a sweet potato, so that's what's called for in this recipe. They're astronomically high in the powerful antioxidant beta-carotene as well as vitamin A.

1 TEASPOON EXTRA-VIRGIN OLIVE OIL

1 SWEET ONION, FINELY DICED

2 TEASPOONS MINCED GARLIC

3 CELERY STALKS, DICED

4 CUPS VEGETABLE STOCK

3 SWEET POTATOES, PEELED AND CUT INTO 1-INCH CUBES

3 CARROTS, PEELED AND DICED

1 RED BELL PEPPER, SEEDED AND DICED

1 (6-OUNCE) CAN LOW-SODIUM TOMATO PASTE

2 CUPS DRY RED LENTILS, RINSED AND PICKED OVER

½ TEASPOON DRIED THYME

½ TEASPOON DRIED BASIL

½ TEASPOON GROUND CUMIN

½ TEASPOON GROUND CORIANDER

FRESHLY GROUND BLACK PEPPER

continued ▶

Lentil and Sweet Potato Stew *continued* ▶

1. In a large saucepan over medium heat, heat the oil and sauté the onion, garlic, and celery until soft, about 5 minutes.

2. Add the stock, sweet potato, carrots, bell pepper, tomato paste, lentils, and herbs, and bring to a boil.

3. Reduce the heat to medium-low and simmer the stew until the sweet potatoes are tender and the flavors are mellow, about 60 minutes.

4. Season with the black pepper and serve hot.

Tomato Chicken Stew

SERVES 6

- SUMMER
- HIGH PROTEIN
- SUPER FOOD

This stew bursts with many flavors and textures, with the rich taste of tomato at the forefront. The sun-dried tomatoes make for a complex flavor profile and add nutrition, especially if you use homemade Balsamic Roasted Tomatoes (see chapter 10). Since tomatoes lose their moisture quickly, drying them is a very good way to preserve their goodness.

1 TABLESPOON EXTRA-VIRGIN OLIVE OIL

4 SKINLESS, BONELESS CHICKEN BREASTS, CUT INTO 2-INCH PIECES

1 ONION, CHOPPED

1 TABLESPOON MINCED GARLIC

1 RED BELL PEPPER, SEEDED AND SLICED THINLY

1 YELLOW BELL PEPPER, SEEDED AND SLICED THINLY

1 CARROT, PEELED AND SLICED INTO THIN DISKS

2 CELERY STALKS, CHOPPED

FRESH JUICE AND RIND OF 1 LEMON

1 CUP LOW-SODIUM CHICKEN STOCK

3 TOMATOES, COARSELY CHOPPED

½ CUP CHOPPED SUN-DRIED OR OVEN-ROASTED TOMATOES

2 TABLESPOONS CHOPPED FRESH BASIL

FRESHLY GROUND BLACK PEPPER

1. Preheat a large skillet over medium heat.

2. Add the oil and chicken, and sauté until lightly browned, 3 to 5 minutes. Transfer the chicken to a large saucepan and set aside.

continued ▶

Tomato Chicken Stew *continued* ▶

3. Drain the excess fat from the skillet and add the onion, garlic, peppers, carrot, and celery. Sauté over medium heat until the vegetables are tender, about 5 minutes.

4. Transfer the vegetables and their juices to the saucepan with the chicken. Add the lemon juice and rind, stock, and tomatoes. Bring the stew to a boil, then reduce heat to medium-low.

5. Cover and simmer for 60 minutes, stirring occasionally.

6. Add the basil and season with the black pepper; cook for another 5 minutes.

7. Serve immediately.

Fish Fennel Stew

SERVES 6

- ■ SUMMER/FALL
- ■ HIGH PROTEIN
- ■ SUPER FOOD

The best kind of fish for this stew is a firm, white fish that's not too oily: halibut, snapper, grouper, and cod are good choices. These fish don't have a strong flavor, which makes this stew perfect for people who don't usually like fish. Ask your fishmonger for boneless cuts, and then check them yourself at home so you don't end up with dangerous fish bones in your food.

6 TOMATOES, CHOPPED

2 CUPS LOW-FAT, LOW-SODIUM CHICKEN BROTH

1 POUND BONELESS, SKINLESS FISH, CUT INTO 1-INCH PIECES

EXTRA-VIRGIN OLIVE OIL FOR THE SKILLET

1 SWEET ONION, CHOPPED

3 CELERY STALKS, CHOPPED

½ FENNEL BULB, CUT INTO THIN STRIPS

2 TEASPOONS MINCED GARLIC

1 TEASPOON RED CHILI FLAKES

1 TABLESPOON CHOPPED FRESH THYME

1. In a large saucepan over medium-high heat, stir together the tomatoes and broth and bring to a boil.

2. Reduce the heat to medium-low and simmer for 5 minutes. Add the fish to the broth mixture and leave at a simmer.

3. In a large skillet over medium heat, heat the oil and sauté the onion, celery, fennel, garlic, and chili flakes until the vegetables have softened, about 10 minutes.

4. Transfer the vegetables to the pot with the fish broth, turn the heat up to medium-high, and cook until the liquid thickens and the fish is cooked, about 15 minutes.

5. Serve topped with the thyme and season to taste.

CHAPTER TWELVE

Main Dishes

Vegetarian Shepherd's Pie

SERVES 6

- ■ SUMMER
- ■ BUDGET-FRIENDLY
- ■ HIGH PROTEIN
- ■ SUPER FOOD

The stew that bubbles under the fluffy potato topping of this dish is incredibly flavorful and can serve as a meal on its own. The navy beans add real body so you won't miss the meat. Navy beans are an excellent source of fiber, which helps lower cholesterol and stabilize blood sugar.

FOR THE MASHED POTATOES:
4 POTATOES, PEELED AND CUT INTO 1-INCH CHUNKS
¼ CUP LOW-FAT, LOW-SODIUM VEGETABLE BROTH
FRESHLY GROUND BLACK PEPPER

FOR THE STEW:
1 TABLESPOON EXTRA-VIRGIN OLIVE OIL
1 TABLESPOON MINCED GARLIC
½ SWEET ONION, CHOPPED
2 CUPS SLICED BUTTON MUSHROOMS
3 CARROTS, PEELED AND SLICED INTO DISKS
2 CUPS CAULIFLOWER FLORETS
1 CUP FRESH OR FROZEN CORN NIBLETS
4 TOMATOES, COARSELY CHOPPED
½ CUP LOW-FAT, LOW-SODIUM VEGETABLE BROTH

1 TEASPOON CHOPPED FRESH THYME

HOT CHILI FLAKES

FRESHLY GROUND BLACK PEPPER

1 CUP DRAINED AND RINSED SODIUM-FREE CANNED NAVY BEANS

To make the mashed potatoes:

1. In a large saucepan, put the potatoes in enough cold water to cover them.

2. Over medium-high heat, bring the water to a boil. Reduce the heat to medium and simmer until the potatoes are fork-tender, about 15 minutes.

3. Drain the potatoes, return them to the pot, and mash them with the broth. Season with the pepper and set aside.

To make the stew:

1. In a large saucepan over medium-high heat, heat the oil. Add the garlic, onion, and mushrooms. Sauté 3 to 4 minutes, until the onions are translucent.

2. Add the carrot, cauliflower, and corn. Sauté until the vegetables are tender, 7 to 10 minutes.

3. Add the tomatoes, broth, and thyme, season with chili flakes, and stir to combine. Season with the black pepper. Bring the stew to a boil, then reduce the heat to medium-low. Simmer until the liquid begins to reduce, about 15 minutes, then remove the pot from the heat.

4. Add the navy beans and stir to mix thoroughly.

To make the pie:

1. Preheat the oven to 350°F.

2. Spoon the stew into a large casserole dish and top with the mashed potatoes.

3. Bake for 35 to 40 minutes, until the stew is bubbling and the potatoes are lightly browned. Serve piping hot.

Egg White Frittata with Whole-Grain Penne

SERVES 4

- SUMMER
- HIGH PROTEIN
- BUDGET-FRIENDLY

The integration of pasta into a frittata makes this recipe unique—and absolutely perfect for Clean Eating, because it combines protein and complex carbohydrates in one tasty dish. It's versatile, too: you can switch up the vegetables to include whatever's in your fridge or on your favorites list. You can make the frittata ahead of time and freeze it quite successfully.

EXTRA-VIRGIN OLIVE OIL FOR THE SKILLET

1 TEASPOON MINCED GARLIC

½ CUP CHOPPED ONION

⅓ CUP DICED RED BELL PEPPER

⅓ CUP DICED YELLOW BELL PEPPER

2 CUPS WHOLE-GRAIN PENNE, COOKED AL DENTE
    PER PACKAGE DIRECTIONS

8 EGG WHITES

¾ CUP LOW-FAT PLAIN GREEK YOGURT

1 TABLESPOON CHOPPED FRESH PARSLEY

2 TEASPOONS CHOPPED FRESH CHIVES

FRESHLY GROUND BLACK PEPPER

1. Preheat the oven to 350°F.

2. Lightly coat a large ovenproof skillet with oil and heat it over medium heat. Sauté the garlic, onion, and bell peppers until lightly caramelized and softened, about 10 minutes.

3. Stir in the cooked penne, distributing it evenly in the skillet. Turn the heat down to low.

4. Whisk the egg whites with the yogurt and add the parsley and chives. Season with the black pepper. Pour the mixture into the skillet. Gently shake the skillet so the eggs mix well with the penne and vegetables.

5. Put the skillet in the oven. Bake the frittata 20 to 30 minutes, until it is set and golden brown.

6. Cut the frittata into quarters and serve.

Pasta and Pepper Primavera

SERVES 6

- SUMMER
- BUDGET-FRIENDLY
- SUPER FOOD

When served on a huge, pretty platter, this dish makes a big impression on guests gathered on a warm summer evening. The snap peas cook very quickly, so add them last or they'll lose their vibrant green color and become grayish. Snap peas are low in fat and high in vitamin K, which means they're good for your heart, help build a healthy immune system, and support strong bones.

1 TABLESPOON EXTRA-VIRGIN OLIVE OIL OR CANOLA OIL

2 TEASPOONS MINCED GARLIC

1 SWEET ONION, CHOPPED

1 RED BELL PEPPER, SEEDED AND CUT INTO THIN STRIPS

1 YELLOW BELL PEPPER, SEEDED AND CUT INTO THIN STRIPS

1 (15-OUNCE) CAN SODIUM-FREE WHITE KIDNEY BEANS, RINSED
    AND DRAINED

FRESH JUICE AND ZEST OF 1 LEMON

½ TEASPOON CRUSHED DRIED THYME

¼ TEASPOON FRESHLY GROUND BLACK PEPPER

¼ TEASPOON CRUSHED RED PEPPER FLAKES

1 CUP SNAP PEAS, TOUGH STRINGS REMOVED

6 OUNCES DRIED WHOLE-WHEAT SPAGHETTI, COOKED AL DENTE PER
    PACKAGE DIRECTIONS

2 TABLESPOONS FRESHLY SHAVED PARMESAN CHEESE

1. In a large skillet over medium heat, heat the oil. Add the garlic, onion, and bell peppers and sauté for 1 minute.

2. Add the beans, lemon juice and zest, thyme, black pepper, and red pepper flakes.

3. Bring liquid to a boil, then reduce the heat to medium-low. Cook uncovered, stirring, for about 5 minutes, until the vegetables are crisp-tender.

4. Add the snap peas and cook for another minute.

5. Remove the vegetables from the heat. Add spaghetti to the skillet. Toss gently to combine.

6. Serve topped with the Parmesan.

Butternut Squash Curry

SERVES 6

- FALL/WINTER
- BUDGET-FRIENDLY
- SUPER FOOD

Butternut squash readily absorbs the flavors of the spices in this dish; you can use more or less curry, cumin, or coriander to suit your taste. When you buy the squash, look for unblemished, firm skin that you can't pierce with your fingernail. If the skin is thin, it means the squash was harvested too young and you won't get the maximum sweetness in the flesh.

1 BUTTERNUT SQUASH, PEELED AND CUT INTO 1-INCH CHUNKS

1 CARROT, PEELED AND DICED

1 SWEET POTATO, PEELED AND CUT INTO 1-INCH CHUNKS

3 TEASPOONS EXTRA-VIRGIN OLIVE OIL

½ ONION, CHOPPED

1 TEASPOON MINCED GARLIC

½ CAULIFLOWER, CUT INTO FLORETS

1 RED BELL PEPPER, SEEDED AND CUT INTO THIN STRIPS

¼ CUP LIGHT COCONUT MILK

1 TABLESPOON CURRY POWDER

1 TEASPOON GROUND CUMIN

½ TEASPOON GROUND CORIANDER

1 CUP 1-INCH GREEN BEAN PIECES

1 BUNCH BASIL LEAVES, CHOPPED FINE, FOR GARNISH

1. Preheat the oven to 325°F.

2. In a medium bowl, toss the squash, carrot, and sweet potato in 1 teaspoon of the oil and spread evenly on a baking sheet. Roast the vegetables until they are soft to the touch, about 20 minutes.

3. In a large saucepan over medium-high heat, heat the remaining 2 teaspoons of olive oil. Add the onion and garlic and sauté until lightly browned, about 5 minutes.

4. Add the cauliflower and bell pepper and sauté for 2 minutes, until softened.

5. Add the roasted squash, carrot, and sweet potato to the saucepan, then stir in the coconut milk and spices. Bring to a boil.

6. Turn the heat down to medium-low and simmer the curry for about 10 minutes, until it is thick and fragrant.

7. Add the green beans and simmer for 1 more minute. Adjust the seasoning to taste with curry and cumin.

8. Serve over brown rice or quinoa, garnished with the basil.

Sea Scallops with Coconut Curry Sauce

SERVES 4

- FALL/WINTER
- QUICK & EASY
- HIGH PROTEIN
- SUPER FOOD

Scallops are one of the easiest mollusks to cook, which is fortunate because they're extremely healthful. An excellent source of vitamin B_{12}, selenium, protein, and omega-3 fats, scallops can significantly benefit the cardiovascular system. When choosing scallops at the fish counter, make sure their flesh is firm and white, and that they have either a faint, sweet scent or no odor at all. Freshness is key when it comes to seafood.

1 POUND SEA SCALLOPS, RINSED AND COMPLETELY DRIED

FRESHLY GROUND BLACK PEPPER

1 TABLESPOON EXTRA-VIRGIN OLIVE OIL

½ ONION, FINELY CHOPPED

2 CARROTS, PEELED AND SLICED INTO THIN DISKS

1 RED BELL PEPPER, SEEDED AND CUT INTO THIN STRIPS

1 YELLOW BELL PEPPER, SEEDED AND CUT INTO THIN STRIPS

1 TABLESPOON FRESHLY GRATED GINGER

1 TEASPOON THAI RED CURRY PASTE

½ CUP LIGHT COCONUT MILK

2 TABLESPOONS CHOPPED FRESH BASIL

FRESH JUICE AND ZEST OF 1 LIME

1. Season the scallops with the pepper.

2. Heat a large nonstick skillet over medium-high heat and add the oil. Put the scallops in the pan and cook them without stirring, until they are browned and crisp on one side, about 3 minutes. Carefully turn the scallops over and sear the other side until browned and crisp, about 3 minutes.

3. Transfer the seared scallops to a serving plate and cover them loosely with foil.

4. Return the skillet to medium heat without cleaning it. Add the onion, carrots, bell peppers, and ginger and sauté for 3 to 4 minutes.

5. Stir in the curry paste and coconut milk and bring the sauce to a simmer, stirring, about 2 minutes. Add the basil, lime juice, and zest and stir to blend.

6. Reduce the heat to low and return the seared scallops to the pan along with any juices on the plate.

7. Turn the scallops to coat them with the sauce. Serve over brown rice.

Clean Tuna Noodle Casserole

SERVES 6

- ■ SUMMER/FALL
- ■ BUDGET-FRIENDLY
- ■ HIGH PROTEIN
- ■ SUPER FOOD

Tuna noodle casserole has suffered a bad reputation, in part because it traditionally features a gooey sauce and a thick topping of crumbled potato chips. By contrast, this variation tastes light and clean and will leave you feeling energized rather than sluggish after eating it. Buy low-sodium rather than regular water-packed canned tuna; it has about 3 percent sodium instead of about 9 percent.

1 TABLESPOON EXTRA-VIRGIN OLIVE OIL

2 CUPS SLICED FRESH MUSHROOMS

¾ CUP CHOPPED ONION

2 CUPS LOW-FAT, LOW-SODIUM CHICKEN BROTH

2 TABLESPOONS ARROWROOT POWDER MIXED WITH ¼ CUP COOL WATER

4 TABLESPOONS GRATED PARMESAN CHEESE

1 TABLESPOON CHOPPED FRESH DILL

6 CUPS COOKED WHOLE-WHEAT ROTINI

1 HEAD BROCCOLI, CUT INTO FLORETS AND LIGHTLY BLANCHED

1 (6-OUNCE) CAN LOW-SODIUM, WATER-PACKED SOLID WHITE OR LIGHT TUNA, DRAINED AND BROKEN INTO CHUNKS

1. Preheat the oven to 325°F.

2. In a large saucepan over medium-high heat, heat the oil and sauté the mushrooms and onion until soft, about 5 minutes.

3. Pour in the broth and bring to a simmer. Turn the heat down to medium-low. Add the arrowroot and whisk for 1 minute, until the sauce thickens.

4. Whisk in the Parmesan and dill and remove from the heat. Add the rotini, broccoli, and tuna and toss to combine thoroughly.

5. Transfer the mixture to a 9-by-13-inch baking dish and bake until the edges are bubbly, about 35 minutes.

Sesame Maple Salmon with Spinach

SERVES 6

- FALL
- QUICK & EASY
- HIGH PROTEIN
- SUPER FOOD

The scent of sesame is so luscious that it imparts incredible richness to other ingredients. When combined with a hint of maple syrup, it can become addictive. Sesame was used extensively for its flavor and medicinal properties more than five thousand years ago. It's extremely high in calcium and magnesium and has been studied extensively as a therapy for several cancers, including leukemia, as well as diabetes and cardiovascular disease.

4 TEASPOONS SESAME SEEDS
6 (6-OUNCE) SALMON FILLETS
FRESHLY GROUND BLACK PEPPER
2 TABLESPOONS PURE MAPLE SYRUP
¼ CUP WATER
2 BUNCHES SPINACH
1 SCALLION, THINLY SLICED ON THE BIAS, FOR GARNISH

1. In a small pan over medium-high heat, toast the sesame seeds while shaking the pan, until they are aromatic and lightly browned. Remove from the heat and set aside.

2. Preheat the oven to 450°F.

3. Place the salmon in a large nonstick baking dish. Season lightly with the pepper, then drizzle with the maple syrup.

4. Bake for 10 to 12 minutes.

5. While the fish is baking, heat a large skillet over medium-high heat and pour in the water. Add the spinach and cook, tossing, until it is bright green.

6. Remove the salmon from the oven, sprinkle with the sesame seeds, and serve with the spinach and garnished with scallion.

Baked Halibut Vegetable Casserole

SERVES 4

- WINTER
- HIGH PROTEIN
- SUPER FOOD

Food for the body and the soul, casseroles provide warm, comforting nourishment that friends and family share from the same dish. This one is packed with wholesome ingredients, such as leeks, which support a healthy cardiovascular system. When preparing leeks, make sure to wash them thoroughly after cutting them, as dirt lodges deeply amid all the layers.

2 CUPS THINLY SLICED CARROT

2 CUPS SLICED FRESH MUSHROOMS

2 LEEKS, SLICED

1 TEASPOON MINCED GARLIC

½ TEASPOON DRIED THYME

¼ TEASPOON FRESHLY GROUND BLACK PEPPER

1 TEASPOON EXTRA-VIRGIN OLIVE OIL

16 BABY POTATOES, BLANCHED AND CUT IN HALF

4 (6-OUNCE) SKINLESS HALIBUT FILLETS

FRESH JUICE OF 2 LEMONS

4 OREGANO SPRIGS (OPTIONAL)

1. Preheat the oven to 350°F.

2. From a roll of heavy foil, tear four 18-by-24-inch pieces. Fold each piece in half to make four 18-by-12-inch pieces.

3. In a large bowl, combine the carrot, mushrooms, leeks, garlic, thyme, pepper, and oil; toss gently.

4. Divide the vegetables among the four pieces of foil, placing them in the center. Top each pile of vegetables with potatoes.

5. Place one piece of fish on each pile and sprinkle with lemon juice. Top with a sprig of oregano (if using).

6. Fold the foil to create sealed packages that have a bit of space for steam to collect. Arrange the halibut packets on a baking pan.

7. Bake for about 30 minutes, until the fish begins to flake.

8. Open the packets carefully, plate, and serve.

Curried Chicken Couscous

SERVES 3

- ■ WINTER
- ■ QUICK & EASY
- ■ HIGH PROTEIN
- ■ SUPER FOOD

Couscous, a form of pasta, has spent some time on the do-not-eat lists of people who avoid carbohydrates. Regular couscous, which is made of refined white flour, should indeed be avoided when eating cleanly, but whole-wheat couscous is a healthful choice. You'll love how quick and simple it is to make!

1 TEASPOON EXTRA-VIRGIN OLIVE OIL

½ SWEET ONION, CHOPPED

1 RED BELL PEPPER, SEEDED AND DICED

1½ CUPS LOW-FAT, LOW-SODIUM CHICKEN BROTH

1 CUP DRY WHOLE-WHEAT COUSCOUS

1 TEASPOON CURRY POWDER

PINCH OF GROUND CINNAMON

½ CUP CHOPPED DRIED APRICOTS

1 CUP DICED, COOKED SKINLESS, BONELESS CHICKEN BREAST

2 SCALLIONS, THINLY SLICED

2 TABLESPOONS SLICED, TOASTED ALMONDS

1. In a large saucepan over medium-low heat, warm the oil. Add the onion and pepper and sauté until the onion is translucent, about 2 minutes.

2. Add the broth, turn the heat up to medium-high, and bring to a boil.

3. Remove the broth from the heat. Add the couscous, curry powder, cinnamon, and apricots and stir to combine. Cover the saucepan and allow it to sit for about 10 minutes.

4. Microwave the chicken breast for about 30 seconds, until it is just warmed.

5. Fluff the cooked couscous with a fork and add the chicken, scallions, and toasted almonds; toss well and serve.

Chicken and Grilled Vegetable Lasagna

SERVES 8

- ■ SUMMER/FALL
- ■ HIGH PROTEIN
- ■ SUPER FOOD

This chicken lasagna is a masterpiece of vibrantly flavored vegetable layers, with just a smattering of cheese. Be sure to reduce the sauce to a thick consistency before you assemble the dish, as watery sauce will result in lasagna that falls apart when you cut it.

1 TABLESPOON PLUS 3 TEASPOONS EXTRA-VIRGIN OLIVE OIL

2 (8-OUNCE) SKINLESS, BONELESS CHICKEN BREASTS

2 RED ONIONS, SLICED INTO DISKS

1 EGGPLANT, CUT INTO 1-INCH-SLICES

1 RED BELL PEPPER, SEEDED AND CUT IN HALF

2 GREEN ZUCCHINI, SLICED LENGTHWISE INTO ½-INCH SLABS

1 YELLOW SUMMER SQUASH, SLICED LENGTHWISE INTO ½-INCH SLABS

1 TABLESPOON MINCED GARLIC

2 CUPS SLICED MUSHROOMS

2 TOMATOES, CHOPPED COARSELY

2 TEASPOONS DRIED BASIL

1 TABLESPOON DRIED OREGANO

PINCH OF RED CHILI FLAKES

1 (16 OUNCE) PACKAGE WHOLE-GRAIN LASAGNA NOODLES, COOKED PER PACKAGE DIRECTIONS

¼ CUP FRESHLY GRATED PARMESAN

continued ▶

1. Preheat the grill or broiler on medium heat.

2. Brush the grill rack or coat the broiler pan with 1 teaspoon or so of the oil. Grill or broil the chicken breasts until cooked through, 2 to 3 minutes per side, and set aside on a clean plate.

3. In a large bowl, toss together 1 tablespoon of oil, red onion, eggplant, bell pepper, and zucchini.

4. Grill or broil the vegetables until tender and lightly charred, about 2 minutes per side. Remove to the plate with the chicken.

5. Let the chicken and vegetables cool slightly, then chop them coarsely.

6. Preheat the oven to 400°F.

7. In a large skillet over medium-high heat, heat the remaining 2 teaspoons of oil. Add the garlic and mushrooms and sauté until soft, about 3 minutes. Stir in the chicken, vegetables, tomatoes, herbs, and chili flakes.

8. Bring the sauce to a boil, then reduce the heat to medium-low and simmer for 10 to 15 minutes, stirring occasionally. All the water should be evaporated. Remove the sauce from the heat.

9. In a deep 9-by-13-inch baking dish, spread a layer of sauce, then a layer of noodles, and repeat until the ingredients are used up, with a layer of sauce on top. Scatter the Parmesan over the top.

10. Bake until the lasagna is bubbly and hot, about 35 minutes.

11. Remove the lasagna from the oven. Allow to cool for 10 to 15 minutes before cutting into 8 servings.

Jambalaya

SERVES 6

- SUMMER
- HIGH PROTEIN
- SUPER FOOD

Shrimp, a traditional ingredient in jambalaya, can be environmentally question-able, but it's perfectly possible to buy good shrimp, whether fresh or frozen, in your supermarket. For health and environmental reasons, avoid shrimp that's farmed in Asia or South America, or that's wild caught by trawlers anywhere in the world. Instead, choose shrimp that's wild caught with traps or that's farmed in the United States, because the U.S. seafood regulations are quite strict. To make your life easier, you can buy shrimp already cleaned, with its shells and veins removed. For this recipe, source out shrimp that are labeled "16/20," which means there are sixteen to twenty per pound and are quite large.

2 SKINLESS, BONELESS CHICKEN BREASTS, CUT INTO STRIPS

FRESHLY GROUND BLACK PEPPER

1 TABLESPOON EXTRA-VIRGIN OLIVE OIL

1 RED ONION, PEELED AND CHOPPED

1 TABLESPOON MINCED GARLIC

1 RED BELL PEPPER, SEEDED AND CHOPPED

1 YELLOW BELL PEPPER, SEEDED AND CHOPPED

3 SCALLIONS, SLICED

2 CUPS LONG-GRAIN BROWN RICE OR ANOTHER FAVORITE WHOLE GRAIN

3 CUPS LOW-FAT, LOW-SODIUM CHICKEN BROTH

SPLASH OF HOT SAUCE

¼ TEASPOON CAYENNE PEPPER

6 (16/20 COUNT) SHRIMP, SHELLED, DEVEINED, AND CHOPPED COARSELY

1. Preheat the oven to 300°F.

2. Season the chicken breast lightly with pepper.

continued ▶

3. In a large, ovenproof skillet over medium-high heat, heat the oil and sauté the chicken until just cooked through, about 3 minutes. Remove the chicken to a clean plate.

4. Do not wipe out the skillet; return it to the heat. Add the onion, garlic, bell peppers, and scallions to the skillet and sauté until tender, about 5 minutes.

5. Add the chicken to the skillet and stir to combine. Add the rice, broth, hot sauce, cayenne, and shrimp.

6. Bring the liquid to a boil, then reduce the heat to medium-low. Simmer for about 5 minutes, stirring constantly.

7. Cover the skillet with a lid and bake for about 45 minutes.

8. Remove the cover and bake an additional 10 minutes.

9. Serve over brown rice.

Chicken and Bulgur Florentine

SERVES 6

- SPRING/SUMMER
- HIGH PROTEIN
- SUPER FOOD

This casserole has lovely colors from the vegetables and wonderful texture from the bulgur. Chewy when cooked, bulgur has a nice nutty taste that pairs well with chicken and spinach. High in fiber and low in fat, it benefits cardiovascular, digestive, and bone health; it can also help prevent cancer and gallstones.

1 TABLESPOON EXTRA-VIRGIN OLIVE OIL

3 (8-OUNCE) SKINLESS, BONELESS CHICKEN BREASTS

2 ONIONS, CHOPPED

1 CUP SLICED FRESH MUSHROOMS

1 TABLESPOON MINCED GARLIC

1 CUP UNCOOKED BULGUR

2 CUPS LOW-FAT, LOW-SODIUM CHICKEN BROTH

½ CUP WATER

¼ TEASPOON GROUND NUTMEG

1 (12-OUNCE) CAN NONFAT EVAPORATED MILK

2 TABLESPOONS ARROWROOT POWDER

4 PACKED CUPS FRESH SPINACH

FRESHLY GROUND BLACK PEPPER

FRESH JUICE AND FINELY SHREDDED PEEL FROM 1 LEMON

1. In a large Dutch oven over medium-high heat, heat the oil. Add the chicken and cook for 12 to 15 minutes, until cooked through.

2. Remove the chicken to a plate and set aside. When the chicken is cool to the touch, chop it coarsely.

continued ▶

3. Add the onions, mushrooms, and garlic to the Dutch oven and sauté for 5 minutes.

4. Stir in the bulgur and stir for 1 minute. Add the broth, water, and nutmeg. Bring the liquid to a boil and reduce the heat to medium-low.

5. Simmer, covered, for 25 to 30 minutes.

6. In a small bowl, whisk together the evaporated milk and arrowroot until smooth.

7. Stir the evaporated milk mixture into the bulgur mixture. Cook, stirring until bubbly and thickened.

8. Stir in the spinach and chicken and simmer for another 5 minutes. Season with the pepper.

9. Serve with a little lemon juice and shredded lemon peel.

Protein-Packed BBQ Beans

SERVES 8

- ■ SUMMER
- ■ BUDGET-FRIENDLY
- ■ HIGH PROTEIN
- ■ SUPER FOOD

Just like the pot of beans you can envision simmering over a campfire on the open range, these beans taste amazing, plus they're packed with protein and fiber. Lean pork, trimmed of excess fat, is a smart choice for anyone eating cleanly. Look for pork from pastured animals that are free to roam outdoors and eat natural foods. The rich flavor of these beans comes partly from tamari, a soy sauce which has little or no wheat (yes, soy sauce contains wheat). Try to find Japanese tamari, which isn't as salty and has a lovely sweetish flavor.

1 TEASPOON EXTRA-VIRGIN OLIVE OIL

½ POUND LEAN GROUND PORK

1 TEASPOON MINCED GARLIC

1 ONION, DICED

1 TABLESPOON DIJON MUSTARD

2 TABLESPOONS TAMARI

⅓ CUP MAPLE SYRUP

¼ CUP LOW-SODIUM TOMATO PASTE

SPLASH OF HOT SAUCE

PINCH OF ALLSPICE

4 (15-OUNCE) CANS SODIUM-FREE NAVY OR WHITE BEANS,
    DRAINED AND RINSED

1. In a medium saucepan over medium-low heat, heat the oil. Add the ground pork and sauté until it is cooked through.

2. Drain off any excess fat and add the minced garlic and onion; sauté until they are translucent.

continued ▶

3. Stir in the mustard and tamari, turn the heat up to medium-high, and bring mixture to a boil.

4. Stir in the maple syrup, tomato paste, hot sauce, and allspice.

5. Bring the sauce back to a boil and cook for 2 minutes.

6. Add the beans to the sauce and simmer for another 5 minutes.

7. Serve in shallow bowls.

Roast Pork Loin with Fennel

SERVES 8

- FALL/WINTER
- BUDGET-FRIENDLY
- HIGH PROTEIN
- LOW-FAT
- SUPER FOOD

You might want to save this spectacular recipe for a special dinner with family and friends. Another great thing about it is that you can make lean, healthful wraps the next day for lunch. Pork has less cholesterol and fat than beef or chicken, and contains eight of the nine essential amino acids along with generous amounts of iron, zinc, and B vitamins. The roast has to be tied up, but you can ask the butcher at your supermarket to do it for you.

2 FENNEL BULBS, FRONDS CUT OFF AND BULBS CUT INTO EIGHTHS

2 TABLESPOONS EXTRA-VIRGIN OLIVE OIL

1 TEASPOON MINCED GARLIC

1 TABLESPOON MAPLE SYRUP

2 POUNDS BONED PORK LOIN, TRIMMED OF VISIBLE FAT

2 TABLESPOONS FENNEL SEEDS

1 TEASPOON FRESHLY GROUND BLACK PEPPER

1 TABLESPOON CHOPPED FRESH THYME

1. Preheat the oven to 375°F.

2. In a large bowl, toss the fennel pieces with 1 tablespoon of oil, garlic, and maple syrup until well coated; set aside.

3. Tie the pork with twine or butcher's string in 4 or 5 places to form a tight cylinder (or have your butcher do it for you).

continued ▶

4. In small bowl, stir together the fennel seeds, pepper, and thyme, then spread the spices out on a plate; set aside.

5. In a large skillet over medium-high heat, heat the remaining 1 tablespoon of oil. Put in the roast and brown it on all sides, about 15 minutes. Remove it from the skillet and allow to cool on a platter.

6. When the roast has cooled, roll it in the herb mixture until evenly coated. Put the meat in large roasting pan and arrange the fennel around the sides.

7. Roast the pork until cooked through but still juicy, about 1½ hours.

8. Transfer the roast and fennel to a serving plate and pour the pan juices over the top. Allow it to rest for 10 minutes before cutting. Slice and serve.

Asian Ginger Pork

SERVES 4

- SUMMER
- HIGH PROTEIN
- SUPER FOOD

The popularity of Asian food makes it fairly easy to find quality Asian season-ings and ingredients that suit a Clean Eating plan. Tamari, a type of soy sauce, contains very little or no wheat and is less salty than regular soy sauce. The Japanese variety is especially good.

1 POUND PORK TENDERLOIN, TRIMMED OF VISIBLE FAT

FRESHLY GROUND BLACK PEPPER

1 TABLESPOON EXTRA-VIRGIN OLIVE OIL

1 TABLESPOON FRESHLY GRATED GINGER

1 TEASPOON MINCED GARLIC

1 TABLESPOON TAMARI

FRESH JUICE AND ZEST OF 1 ORANGE

½ CUP LOW-FAT, LOW-SODIUM VEGETABLE BROTH

3 SCALLIONS, SLICED THINLY

½ RED BELL PEPPER, SEEDED AND CUT INTO VERY THIN STRIPS

1. Preheat the oven to 400°F.

2. Season the pork lightly all over with the pepper.

3. Heat a large ovenproof skillet over medium-high heat and add the oil. Brown the pork on all sides.

4. Put the skillet in the oven and roast the pork for 20 minutes, or until just cooked through. Remove the meat to a plate and cover with foil to keep warm.

continued ▶

5. Do not clean the pan; place it on medium heat. Add the ginger and garlic to the skillet and sauté for 1 minute, then add the tamari, orange juice and zest, and broth.

6. Simmer the sauce for 15 minutes and remove from heat.

7. Stir in the scallions and bell pepper to coat.

8. Slice the pork into 1-inch slices and toss them with the sauce, along with any juices from the plate.

9. Serve over brown rice or your favorite whole grain.

Herb-Crusted Pork Chops

SERVES 4

- ■ SUMMER/FALL
- ■ BUDGET-FRIENDLY
- ■ HIGH PROTEIN
- ■ SUPER FOOD

To make this dish the very best it can be, it's crucial to use fresh, ideally organic, herbs. Your supermarket probably carries herbs in sealed plastic containers or you can buy them loose, choosing the most fragrant bunches: lightly bruise a couple of leaves to release the essential oils and get a good whiff. Of course, it's even better to grow your own herbs, if possible.

4 TEASPOONS DIJON MUSTARD

4 BONELESS PORK CHOPS, TRIMMED OF VISIBLE FAT

½ CUP WHOLE-WHEAT BREADCRUMBS

2 TEASPOONS CHOPPED FRESH THYME

1 TEASPOON CHOPPED FRESH PARSLEY

¼ TEASPOON CHOPPED FRESH ROSEMARY

PINCH OF FRESHLY GROUND BLACK PEPPER

2 TEASPOONS EXTRA-VIRGIN OLIVE OIL

1. Preheat the oven to 450°F.

2. Line a baking dish with foil and set aside.

3. Rub 1 teaspoon of the mustard over each pork chop, coating both sides.

4. In a small bowl, combine the breadcrumbs, herbs, and pepper; spread out the mixture on a plate. Lightly dredge each chop in the breadcrumb mixture.

5. In a large skillet over medium-high heat, heat the oil. Place the chops in the skillet and brown them on both sides.

6. Put the chops in the baking dish and bake for about 8 minutes, or until the pork reaches 145°F in the center.

7. Let the chops rest for 5 minutes before serving.

Beef Sirloin Kebabs in Herb Garlic Marinade

SERVES 4

- ■ SUMMER/FALL
- ■ QUICK & EASY
- ■ HIGH PROTEIN
- ■ SUPER FOOD

Beef has long been considered to be a great protein for power lifters and body-builders, but select red meat with care. Look for organic, pastured, 100 percent grass-fed beef, preferably from a local farm. If you don't have access to this kind of meat, seek out the most healthful beef available at your supermarket: try to avoid antibiotics, added hormones, and steroids.

2 GARLIC CLOVES, CHOPPED

1 TABLESPOON CHOPPED FRESH THYME

1 TABLESPOON CHOPPED FRESH ROSEMARY

2 TABLESPOONS RED WINE VINEGAR

1 TABLESPOON LOW-SODIUM SOY SAUCE

1 TABLESPOON EXTRA-VIRGIN OLIVE OIL, PLUS MORE FOR THE GRILL

1 TEASPOON FRESHLY GROUND BLACK PEPPER

1 POUND BONELESS TOP SIRLOIN STEAK, TRIMMED OF VISIBLE FAT AND CUT INTO 2-INCH CHUNKS

1 RED ONION, QUARTERED AND SEPARATED INTO LAYERS

1 RED BELL PEPPER, SEEDED AND CUT INTO 1½-INCH CHUNKS

1 YELLOW BELL PEPPER, SEEDED AND CUT INTO 1½-INCH CHUNKS

1 GREEN BELL PEPPER, SEEDED AND CUT INTO 1½-INCH CHUNKS

4 WOODEN SKEWERS

1. In a large bowl, stir together the garlic, thyme, rosemary, vinegar, soy sauce, 1 tablespoon oil, and ½ teaspoon of black pepper until well blended.

2. Add the beef and stir to coat.

3. Cover the bowl and refrigerate for 6 to 12 hours, stirring occasionally. When you're ready to make the kebabs, put the skewers in water to soak for 30 minutes.

4. Heat the grill to medium-high.

5. Remove the beef from the refrigerator and assemble the kebabs, alternating pieces of beef, onion, and bell pepper on the skewers.

6. Sprinkle the kebabs with remaining ½ teaspoon of black pepper.

7. Lightly brush the grill rack with olive oil.

8. Grill the kebabs, turning once or twice, until the beef is done, 6 to 8 minutes for medium-rare or 9 to 11 minutes for medium.

9. Transfer the kebabs to a plate and let them rest for 5 minutes before serving.

Baked Stuffed Tomatoes

SERVES 4

- SUMMER
- BUDGET-FRIENDLY
- SUPER FOOD

Stuffing vegetables is an efficient way to present striking, healthful meals without any muss or fuss. Tomatoes are particularly good because they impart a great deal of juicy flavor to the filling. Low in everything you should avoid in your diet—sodium, cholesterol, saturated fat, calories—tomatoes are a fine source of fiber, B vitamins, and copper. Pick firm but ripe tomatoes that are big enough to hold about three-fourths cup of filling.

2 TABLESPOONS EXTRA-VIRGIN OLIVE OIL, PLUS MORE
    FOR THE BAKING DISH
8 FIRM, RIPE TOMATOES, ABOUT 3 INCHES IN DIAMETER
2 CUPS COOKED BROWN RICE
1 CUP COOKED, EXTRA-LEAN GROUND BEEF
1 GREEN PEPPER, SEEDED AND DICED
½ ONION, CHOPPED
⅓ CUP CHOPPED FRESH BASIL
2 TEASPOONS MINCED GARLIC
FRESHLY GROUND BLACK PEPPER
2 TABLESPOONS FRESHLY GRATED PARMESAN CHEESE

1. Preheat the oven to 375°F.

2. Lightly oil a shallow 9-by-13-inch baking dish and set aside.

3. Cut about ½ inch off the top of each tomato and set the tops aside.

4. Carefully scoop the pulp out of the tomatoes, leaving as thick a shell as possible. Separate as many seeds out as possible from the pulp and discard. Chop up the pulp.

5. In a large bowl, stir together the rice, beef, pepper, onion, basil, garlic, 1 tablespoon of oil, and about ½ cup of the tomato pulp. Season with the pepper.

6. Arrange the tomato shells in the baking dish. Spoon the rice mixture into the tomatoes and sprinkle with the Parmesan.

7. Cover the filled tomatoes with their tops and drizzle with the remaining 1 tablespoon of oil. Bake for 15 to 20 minutes, basting with the juices, until the tomatoes are soft to the touch.

8. Serve 2 tomatoes on each plate, warm or at room temperature.

Balsamic-Marinated Beef Roast

SERVES 6

- ■ WINTER/SPRING
- ■ QUICK & EASY
- ■ HIGH PROTEIN
- ■ LOW-SODIUM

One of the ingredients in this savory marinade might seem like an afterthought rather than an essential component. This humble ingredient is black pepper. In many recipes, it's casually sprinkled on "to taste" rather than as a main flavoring, but it can add extra dimension when it's more prominent. It might surprise you that black pepper can aid your digestion. When it stimulates your taste buds, it signals your stomach to produce hydrochloric acid, lessening the likelihood of indigestion.

⅓ CUP BALSAMIC VINEGAR

3 TEASPOONS MINCED GARLIC

1 TEASPOON CHOPPED FRESH THYME

1 TEASPOON GROUND DRIED ROSEMARY

2 TABLESPOONS EXTRA-VIRGIN OLIVE OIL

1 TEASPOON FRESHLY GROUND BLACK PEPPER

1 (2-POUND) BONELESS SIRLOIN TOP ROAST

1. In a large bowl, whisk together all the ingredients except the roast until well blended.

2. Add the meat, turn it to coat evenly with the marinade, and cover the bowl with plastic wrap.

3. Put the roast in the fridge and marinate for 4 to 18 hours, turning several times.

4. Preheat the oven to 450°F.

5. Put the meat on a rack in a roasting pan and roast for 15 minutes. Reduce the heat to 275°F.

6. Continue roasting until the meat reaches the doneness you desire: an internal temperature of 120°F to 125°F for rare, about 45 minutes; 130°F to 135°F for medium rare, about 50 minutes; and 140°F to 145°F for medium, about 60 minutes.

7. Remove the roast from the oven and allow it to rest for 10 minutes before carving.

Herbed Beef Burgers

SERVES 6

- ■ SUMMER/FALL
- ■ QUICK & EASY
- ■ BUDGET-FRIENDLY
- ■ HIGH PROTEIN
- ■ SUPER FOOD

Served at barbecues, casual family dinners, sporting events, and picnics, hamburgers are a huge part of summer. They don't usually rank high on healthful food lists, but it's actually the toppings and bun that give them the bad reputation. This recipe is so savory and juicy that you won't even miss the fattening stuff!

1 POUND EXTRA-LEAN GROUND BEEF

⅓ CUP OAT FLOUR

¼ CUP SHREDDED CARROT

¼ CUP CHOPPED RED ONION

2 EGG WHITES, LIGHTLY BEATEN

1 TEASPOON CHOPPED FRESH THYME

½ TEASPOON CHOPPED FRESH ROSEMARY

½ TEASPOON CHOPPED FRESH OREGANO

PINCH OF FRESHLY GROUND BLACK PEPPER

1 SMALL TOMATO, SLICED

½ AVOCADO, PEELED, PITTED, AND CHOPPED

6 MULTIGRAIN BUNS

1. Preheat the grill to medium-high.

2. In a large bowl, thoroughly mix together the beef, flour, carrot, onion, egg whites, and spices with your hands.

3. Divide the mixture into 6 equal balls and flatten them between your hands into burgers.

4. Grill the burgers until cooked through but still juicy, flipping once, about 7 minutes per side.

5. Top each burger with fresh tomato and diced avocado, and serve on a multigrain bun or on its own.

CHAPTER THIRTEEN

Desserts

Traditional Apple Crisp

SERVES 8

- FALL
- QUICK & EASY
- HIGH PROTEIN
- SUPER FOOD

This dessert is usually made with lots of butter and brown sugar, but this version uses apple butter to both bind and sweeten the crisp top of the dish. Apple butter is a wonderful source of insoluble fiber, vitamin A, and vitamin C. This means it's great for digestive health and can reduce your risk of colon cancer.

3 TABLESPOONS CHIA SEEDS (SEE THE GLOSSARY)

½ CUP UNSWEETENED APPLE JUICE

EXTRA-VIRGIN OLIVE OIL FOR THE BAKING DISH

6 TART APPLES, PEELED, CORED, AND SLICED THIN

4 TABLESPOONS APPLE BUTTER

1 CUP LARGE-FLAKE OATS

1 TEASPOON GROUND CINNAMON

½ TEASPOON GROUND NUTMEG

¼ TEASPOON GROUND CLOVES

PINCH OF SEA SALT

1. In a small bowl, whisk the chia seeds and apple juice together and set aside for at least 4 hours.

2. Preheat the oven to 325°F.

3. Lightly oil a 9-by-9-inch baking dish.

4. Add the apple slices to the apple juice mixture and toss to combine. Spoon the apples into the prepared baking dish.

5. In a large bowl, stir together the apple butter, oats, spices, and salt until crumbly.

6. Top the apples with the oat mixture and bake, covered with aluminum foil, for 25 minutes.

7. Remove the foil and continue to bake for another 15 minutes, until the topping is lightly browned and the apples are bubbly.

Baked Apples

SERVES 6

- FALL
- BUDGET-FRIENDLY
- SUPER FOOD

Part of the delectable sweetness of this dish comes from low-fat, energy-packed raisins. Raisins are a good source of boron, which is critical for bone health, particularly for women who are susceptible to bone loss.

¼ CUP RAISINS

½ CUP ROLLED OATS

3 TABLESPOONS ALMOND BUTTER, MICROWAVED
    IN 10-SECOND INTERVALS UNTIL MELTED

2 TABLESPOONS UNSWEETENED APPLE JUICE

1 TABLESPOON MAPLE SYRUP

6 TART APPLES, CORED

½ TEASPOON GROUND CINNAMON

½ TEASPOON GROUND NUTMEG

1. Preheat the oven to 350°F.

2. In a large bowl, stir together the raisins and oats.

3. In a small bowl, combine the almond butter, apple juice, and maple syrup.

4. Spoon the oat mixture into the cored apples and place them in a 9-by-13-inch baking dish.

5. Sprinkle the stuffed apples with the spices, and spoon the almond butter mixture over the top.

6. Cover the baking dish with a lid or aluminum foil and cook the apples until tender, 35 to 45 minutes.

Grilled Pineapple with Cinnamon Yogurt Sauce

SERVES 6

- SPRING/SUMMER
- QUICK & EASY
- BUDGET-FRIENDLY
- LOW-FAT
- SUPER FOOD

Pineapple is available year-round, but it's particularly sweet and bright-hued from March to July. It's high in vitamin C and manganese, helping reduce your risk of cardiovascular disease and cancer. Unlike other fruit, pineapple doesn't keep ripening once it's harvested, so it's important to buy the ripest one you can find and store it in the fridge until you want to use it. To determine ripeness, choose one that is golden in color rather than greenish.

EXTRA-VIRGIN OLIVE OIL FOR THE GRILL

1 CUP NONFAT PLAIN GREEK YOGURT

2 TABLESPOONS HONEY

1 TEASPOON GROUND CINNAMON

1 PINEAPPLE, SKINNED, CORED, AND SLICED INTO
    1-INCH SLICES

1. Preheat the grill to medium heat.

2. Lightly oil the grill.

3. In a small bowl, stir together the yogurt, honey, and cinnamon; set aside.

4. Lay the pineapple slices on the grill and cook for 3 minutes.

5. Flip the pineapple over and grill for another 3 minutes.

6. Arrange the pineapple on 6 plates and serve drizzled with the honey yogurt.

Banana Coconut Soft-Serve Ice Cream

SERVES 6

- ANY SEASON
- QUICK & EASY
- LOW-SODIUM
- BUDGET-FRIENDLY
- SUPER FOOD

This isn't really soft-serve ice cream, but the texture is so close that you won't miss the processed kind. The trick to bringing out the intense, sweet flavor is to make sure your bananas are ripe but still firm when you freeze them. If they're too ripe, the dessert will be runny rather than creamy and thick.

6 BANANAS
1 (13.5-OUNCE) CAN LIGHT COCONUT MILK
¾ CUP UNSWEETENED SHREDDED COCONUT

1. Peel and slice the bananas.

2. Put the banana chunks in a large container and freeze overnight.

3. Transfer the frozen banana to a food processor or blender and process with the coconut milk until smooth and creamy.

4. Serve immediately, topped with the shredded coconut.

Pumpkin Chocolate Cake

SERVES 6

- FALL
- BUDGET-FRIENDLY
- SUPER FOOD

This delectable, moist cake is perfect for a birthday or holiday. Cocoa is an excellent source of minerals, antioxidants, and phytonutrients, and can help in the production of mood-enhancing hormones. Studies have suggested that it may play a role in reducing the risk of cancer, treating heart disease, and lowering high blood pressure. Always buy good-quality cocoa—organic, if possible.

EXTRA-VIRGIN OLIVE OIL FOR THE BAKING DISH

¾ CUP WHOLE-WHEAT PASTRY FLOUR

¾ CUP ALMOND FLOUR

¼ CUP UNSWEETENED COCOA POWDER

1 TABLESPOON BAKING SODA

1 TABLESPOON GROUND CINNAMON

½ TEASPOON GROUND NUTMEG

⅛ TEASPOON SEA SALT

1 CUP CANNED PUMPKIN (NOT PUMPKIN PIE MIX)

¾ CUP HONEY

1 EGG, LIGHTLY BEATEN

2 EGG WHITES, LIGHTLY BEATEN

1 TEASPOON PURE VANILLA EXTRACT

1. Preheat the oven to 350°F.

2. Lightly coat a deep 8-by-8-inch baking dish with the oil.

3. In a medium bowl, stir together the flours, cocoa powder, baking soda, cinnamon, nutmeg, and salt.

continued ▶

Pumkin Chocolate Cake *continued* ▶

4. In a large bowl, stir together the pumpkin, honey, egg, egg whites, and vanilla until well mixed.

5. Add the dry ingredients to the wet ingredients and stir until combined.

6. Spoon the batter into the baking dish and bake for 40 minutes, or until a toothpick inserted in the center comes out clean.

7. Cool on a wire rack, cut into pieces, and serve warm.

Peach Cobbler

SERVES 6

- SUMMER/FALL
- BUDGET-FRIENDLY
- SUPER FOODS

This fresh, sweet dessert really bursts with plump, golden peaches. The fruit needs to be ripe, so choose peaches that have red skin and feel soft to the touch, without being mushy. Ripe peaches have a heady scent that will remind you of warm summer breezes.

EXTRA-VIRGIN OLIVE OIL FOR THE BAKING DISH

1½ CUPS OAT FLOUR

3 TEASPOONS BAKING POWDER

2 EGGS, LIGHTLY BEATEN

⅓ CUP HONEY

½ CUP ALMOND MILK

3 CUPS SLICED PEACHES

1. Preheat the oven to 350°F.

2. Lightly coat a deep 9-by-9-inch baking dish with the oil.

3. In a large bowl, stir together all the ingredients except the peaches, until well combined.

4. Put the peaches in the baking dish. Top the peaches with the cobbler batter.

5. Bake for 35 to 40 minutes, until the top of the cobbler is golden brown.

6. Allow to cool slightly, and serve warm.

Pumpkin Pie Puddings

SERVES 6

- FALL
- QUICK & EASY
- BUDGET-FRIENDLY
- SUPER FOOD

If you love pumpkin pie, this Clean Eating version will be your new favorite treat. It's cooked in a water bath, so when the batter firms up, it remains creamy and doesn't crack. This isn't an overly sweet recipe; add a couple more tablespoons of honey if you like. Honey is known as a powerful antibacterial and antiseptic, so it's good for the digestion and helps combat heartburn.

1 CUP CANNED PUMPKIN (NOT PUMPKIN PIE MIX)
2 TABLESPOONS HONEY
2 EGG WHITES, LIGHTLY BEATEN
½ TEASPOON GROUND CINNAMON
¼ TEASPOON GROUND GINGER
⅛ TEASPOON GROUND CLOVES
1 CUP UNSWEETENED ALMOND MILK

1. Preheat the oven to 425°F.

2. Put six 4-ounce ramekins in a baking dish.

3. Combine all the ingredients in a large mixing bowl and whisk to blend well.

4. Pour the mixture evenly into the ramekins.

5. Add water to the baking dish to reach about 1 inch up the sides of the ramekins, taking care not to get any water in the batter.

6. Bake for 15 minutes, then reduce the heat to 350°F.

7. Bake for 30 to 35 more minutes, until the puddings are set.

8. Remove from the oven and cool completely.

Cherry Granita

SERVES 4

- SUMMER
- QUICK & EASY
- BUDGET-FRIENDLY
- SUPER FOOD

This snowy sweet treat feels like tiny flavored ice crystals on your tongue. Cherries, a very rich source of antioxidants, can help fight cancer and relieve the pain associated with gout, migraines, and arthritis. Cherries can even help you sleep: They increase melatonin levels in the blood.

½ CUP UNSWEETENED APPLE JUICE
¼ CUP HONEY
2 TABLESPOONS FRESHLY SQUEEZED LEMON JUICE
2 CUPS PITTED FRESH CHERRIES

1. Put all the ingredients in a food processor or blender and pulse until well blended.

2. Pour the mixture into a shallow metal baking dish and put the dish in the freezer.

3. Stir the mixture with a fork every 10 to 15 minutes, until it becomes slushy, about 35 minutes.

4. Once the granita is slushy, leave it in the freezer and scrape it around every 5 minutes until it has a crystalized, icy texture.

5. Spoon into cups and serve immediately.

Smooth Lime Pudding

SERVES 6

- ■ SUMMER/FALL
- ■ QUICK & EASY
- ■ BUDGET-FRIENDLY
- ■ SUPER FOOD

The velvety texture of this dessert comes from avocado, which also makes the pudding a pretty, pale green. You can use lemons instead of limes, and the pudding will still be green! Avocado, also called alligator pear, is one of the most nutritious foods on the planet, containing twenty essential nutrients, including omega-3 fatty acids. It has been linked to reduced diabetes risk and improvements in patients suffering from diabetes, Alzheimer's disease, cardiovascular disease, and cancer.

FRESH JUICE OF 2 LIMES
1 TABLESPOON LIME ZEST
4 TABLESPOONS HONEY
2 AVOCADOS, PEELED, PITTED, AND CHOPPED INTO CHUNKS
1 CUP NONFAT PLAIN GREEK YOGURT

1. Put all the ingredients into a food processor or blender and process until completely smooth.

2. Adjust the tartness and spoon into 6 dessert dishes.

Chocolate Pots Crème

SERVES 8

- ■ ANY SEASON
- ■ QUICK & EASY
- ■ SUPER FOOD

Dark chocolate makes a lovely treat when you're eating cleanly—it's not only delicious, but also healthful. Good for the heart and brain, it helps control blood sugar, promotes a healthy immune system, and can even help harden your teeth. Purchase very good quality dark chocolate, organic when possible, because lesser products are highly processed and contain junk fillers such as corn syrup, preservatives, refined sugar, and processed milk powder.

3 CUPS COCONUT MILK
10 OUNCES 70 PERCENT DARK CHOCOLATE,
    FINELY CHOPPED
¼ CUP MAPLE SYRUP
1 TABLESPOON ORANGE ZEST
1 TEASPOON PURE VANILLA EXTRACT

1. Place a medium saucepan over medium heat and bring the coconut milk to a simmer. Remove the milk from the heat.

2. Put the chopped chocolate in a food processor or blender and pour in the hot coconut milk. Add the maple syrup, orange zest, and vanilla extract and process until the chocolate is melted and the mixture is smooth.

3. Pour the mixture through a fine-mesh sieve into a bowl, and spoon it into 8 small ramekins.

4. Cover the ramekins and refrigerate until set, about 3 hours.

Clean Strawberry Cheesecake

SERVES 4

- SPRING/SUMMER
- QUICK & EASY
- SUPER FOOD

Cheesecake: the word itself invokes images of heavenly indulgence. Just thinking about the creaminess, richness, smooth texture, and silky perfection of a perfect cheesecake can add pounds! This dessert has all of cheesecake's sublime qualities, without the excess sugar and fat. If you want a slightly sweeter topping than simple chopped strawberries, you can mix them with a couple tablespoons of sugar-free preserves.

½ CUP NONFAT CREAM CHEESE

2 TABLESPOONS HONEY

½ CUP LOW-FAT PLAIN GREEK YOGURT

1 TABLESPOON FRESHLY SQUEEZED LEMON JUICE

4 DATES

½ CUP COARSELY GROUND ALMONDS

1 CUP FINELY DICED STRAWBERRIES

1. Using a hand beater in a medium bowl, cream together the cream cheese, honey, yogurt, and lemon juice until very smooth. Cover and refrigerate.

2. Put the dates in a food processor or blender and pulse until they're chopped. Add the ground almonds and pulse until combined with the dates.

3. Press the date-almond mixture evenly into the bottoms of 4 ramekins.

4. Spoon the cheesecake filling into the ramekins and top with diced strawberries.

5. Refrigerate for 3 to 4 hours until firm. Serve chilled.

Lemon Frozen Yogurt

MAKES 4 CUPS

- SPRING/SUMMER
- QUICK & EASY
- HIGH PROTEIN
- SUPER FOOD

Much loved around the world, the tart taste of lemon tempts even people who dislike desserts. This smooth, icy treat has a bold lemony taste with just a touch of sweetness. Try to purchase organic lemons because you're going to use the zest, and commercially grown lemons are usually coated with a protective layer of wax. If you can't get organic fruit, use a soft-bristle brush to scrub the wax off the lemons.

¾ CUP HONEY

1 CUP FRESHLY SQUEEZED LEMON JUICE

3 CUPS VANILLA OR PLAIN LOW-FAT GREEK YOGURT

1 TABLESPOON LEMON ZEST

1. In a small saucepan, whisk together the honey and lemon juice. Over medium-high heat, bring the mixture to a boil, then reduce the heat to medium-low and simmer for several minutes, stirring constantly.

2. Remove the mixture from the heat, pour it into a large bowl, and cool completely in the fridge.

3. When the lemon juice mixture is cool, whisk in the yogurt and zest until well blended.

4. Freeze in an ice cream maker according to the manufacturer's instructions.

5. Scoop into bowls and serve cold.

Plum Peach Sorbet

MAKES 4 CUPS

- ■ SUMMER/FALL
- ■ QUICK & EASY
- ■ BUDGET-FRIENDLY
- ■ SUPER FOOD

Black plums are a decadent fruit with rich juice and deep purple flesh that's sweet and tart all at once. They're a great choice for anyone with iron deficiencies, as their abundant vitamin C helps your body absorb iron. When you take this luscious sorbet out of the freezer, let it sit at room temperature for five to ten minutes before serving so that it's easier to scoop.

1 CUP PITTED, SLICED BLACK PLUMS
3 CUPS PITTED, PEELED, AND SLICED PEACHES
1 TEASPOON FRESHLY SQUEEZED LEMON JUICE
¼ CUP HONEY
½ CUP UNSWEETENED APPLE JUICE

1. In a large bowl, stir together the plums, peaches, lemon juice, and honey until the fruit slices are well coated.

2. Transfer the fruit mixture to a food processor or blender and process with the apple juice until very smooth.

3. Pour the liquid into a container and cover it. Chill until the sorbet is completely frozen, about 6 hours.

Slow Cooker Chocolate Cake

MAKES 8 SERVINGS

- ANY SEASON
- QUICK & EASY
- BUDGET-FRIENDLY
- SUPER FOOD

Who says you can't have chocolate cake when eating cleanly? This moist, delicious dessert would be perfect combined with ripe strawberries or a scoop of banana ice cream. Remember to put the oil or parchment paper in the bottom of your slow-cooker insert or it will be impossible to get the cake out.

EXTRA-VIRGIN OLIVE OIL FOR THE SLOW-COOKER INSERT

½ CUP WHOLE-WHEAT PASTRY FLOUR

½ CUP ALMOND FLOUR

½ CUP UNSWEETENED COCOA POWDER

2 TEASPOONS BAKING POWDER

1 CUP UNSWEETENED APPLE SAUCE

½ CUP ALMOND BUTTER

½ CUP HONEY

2 EGG WHITES, LIGHTLY BEATEN

1 TABLESPOON PURE VANILLA EXTRACT

1. Cut a piece of parchment paper (if using) to fit the bottom of your slow cooker and press it in. Very lightly coat the parchment and sides of the slow cooker with oil.

2. In a large bowl, mix together the flours, cocoa powder, and baking powder until well blended.

3. In a medium bowl, beat together the apple sauce, almond butter, honey, egg whites, and vanilla until combined.

continued ▶

4. Add the applesauce mixture to the dry ingredients and stir together well.

5. Spoon the batter into the slow cooker and turn it on low heat. Cook on low for 3 to 4 hours or until a toothpick inserted in the center comes out clean.

6. To remove the cake, simply run a knife around the edges, and allow the cake to cool about 10 minutes in the insert. Then, using oven mitts, cover the insert with a plate and turn it over; the cake will pop right out. Peel off the parchment paper.

7. Cut the cake into squares and serve warm.

Almond Fudge Cups

MAKES 24 CANDIES

- ANY SEASON
- QUICK & EASY
- SUPER FOOD

These may not come in an orange wrapper, but they're as good as peanut butter cups and have none of the added preservatives, flavorings, or sugar. This is a tiny dessert to be enjoyed with a nice cup of coffee while chatting with friends after a festive meal. For a firm texture, make sure to keep these delectable bites in the freezer, since coconut oil is a liquid at room temperature.

1 CUP COCONUT OIL
1 CUP UNSWEETENED COCOA POWDER
1½ CUPS ALMOND BUTTER
½ CUP MAPLE SYRUP
1 TEASPOON PURE VANILLA EXTRACT

1. Arrange 24 foil-lined candy cups in a baking dish and set aside.

2. In a small saucepan over low heat, melt the coconut oil. Transfer to a food processor or blender and add the remaining ingredients. Process until completely blended.

3. Pour the fudge batter into the candy cups until about ¾ full.

4. Put the cups in the freezer for about 60 minutes to set.

5. Store in a sealed container in the freezer.

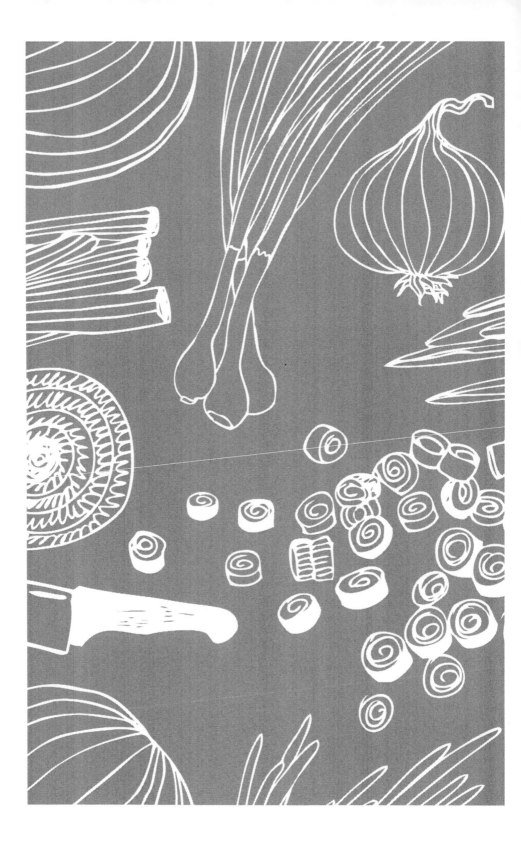

APPENDIX

Clean Eating Food List

Poultry, Meats, and Fish/Seafood

- Bass
- Beef, extra-lean ground
- Beef, grass-fed, trimmed of visible fat
- Buffalo/bison
- Chicken, lean ground
- Chicken breast, skinless, boneless
- Clams
- Crab
- Elk
- Halibut
- Lamb, lean ground
- Lamb, rack
- Lobster
- Mussels
- Pork, lean ground
- Pork chops, trimmed of visible fat
- Pork roast, trimmed of visible fat
- Pork tenderloin
- Salmon, fresh or low-sodium, water-packed canned
- Scallops
- Shrimp
- Tilapia
- Tuna, fresh or low-sodium, water-packed canned
- Turkey, extra-lean ground
- Turkey breast, skinless, boneless
- Veal
- Venison steaks
- Venison tenderloin

Protein Alternatives

- Black beans
- Black-eyed peas
- Chickpeas
- Edamame
- Eggs, organic, free-range
- Kidney beans
- Lentils
- Navy beans
- Split peas
- Tempeh
- Tofu

Vegetables

- Artichokes
- Asparagus
- Beets, beet greens
- Bell peppers
- Broccoli
- Brussels sprouts
- Cabbage
- Carrots
- Cauliflower
- Celeriac/celery root
- Celery
- Chard
- Collard greens
- Cucumbers
- Eggplants
- Garlic
- Green beans
- Greens, dark leafy
- Greens, salad
- Jicama
- Kale
- Leeks
- Mushrooms
- Onions
- Parsnips
- Peas
- Potatoes
- Pumpkin
- Radishes
- Scallions/green onions
- Shallots
- Snap peas
- Snow peas
- Spinach
- Sprouts
- Squash, summer
- Squash, winter
- Sweet potatoes
- Tomatoes, fresh or low-sodium canned
- Turnips
- Watercress
- Wax beans
- Yams
- Zucchini

Fruits

- Apples
- Apricots
- Avocados
- Bananas
- Berries, fresh or frozen
- Cantaloupe
- Cherries
- Dates
- Dried fruit, unsulfured, unsweetened
- Grapefruit
- Grapes
- Figs
- Honeydew melons
- Kiwi
- Lemons
- Limes
- Mangoes
- Nectarines
- Oranges

- Papayas
- Peaches
- Pears
- Pineapples
- Plums
- Pomegranates
- Raisins
- Tangerines
- Watermelon

Dairy and Dairy Alternatives

- Almond milk
- Butter, unsalted
- Cashew milk
- Coconut milk
- Cottage cheese, low-fat or nonfat
- Cream cheese, nonfat
- Feta, low-sodium
- Greek yogurt, low-fat or nonfat plain
- Kefir (yogurt drink)
- Rice milk
- Skim milk
- Soy milk
- Yogurt, low-fat or nonfat plain

Beverages

- Coffee
- Tea, green or herbal
- Water

Nuts, Seeds, and Oil

- Almonds, unsalted
- Avocado oil
- Cashews, unsalted
- Chestnuts
- Chia seeds
- Coconut oil
- Coconut, unsweetened shredded
- Flaxseed
- Hazelnuts, unsalted
- Nut and seed butters, unsalted
- Olive oil
- Pecans, unsalted
- Pine nuts/pignolias
- Pistachios, unsalted, undyed
- Pumpkin seeds/pepitas
- Safflower oil
- Sesame oil
- Sesame seeds, unsalted
- Sunflower seeds, unsalted
- Walnuts, unsalted

Baked Goods

- Brown-rice wraps
- Wasa crispbreads
- Whole-grain breads, pitas, tortillas
- Whole-wheat breadcrumbs

Cereals

- Cold and hot cereal, whole-grain
- Granola, homemade or unsweetened
- Oat bran
- Oatmeal
- Wheat germ

Grains

- Barley
- Buckwheat
- Bulgur
- Millet
- Quinoa
- Rice, brown, wild
- Teff
- Wheat berries

Dry Goods

- Baking powder
- Baking soda
- Black pepper/peppercorns
- Brown rice cakes
- Cocoa powder, unsweetened
- Protein powder, all-natural, unsweetened whey
- Sea salt
- Soba noodles
- Spices (cinnamon, cloves, allspice, cumin, coriander, curry, nutmeg)
- Vanilla extract, pure
- Whole-grain flours (wholewheat, oat, quinoa, amaranth, spelt)
- Whole-grain pasta

Sweeteners

- Agave nectar
- Honey
- Maple syrup
- Stevia

Fresh Herbs

- Basil
- Bay
- Chives
- Cilantro
- Dill
- Lemon balm
- Marjoram
- Mint
- Oregano
- Parsley
- Rosemary
- Sage
- Savory
- Tarragon
- Thyme

Miscellaneous

- Applesauce, unsweetened
- Broth, low-fat, low-sodium vegetable, beef, or chicken
- Hot sauce
- Ketchup, organic
- Mustard
- Olives
- Salsa
- Tahini/sesame butter
- Tamari
- Tomato sauce
- Vinegar, apple cider

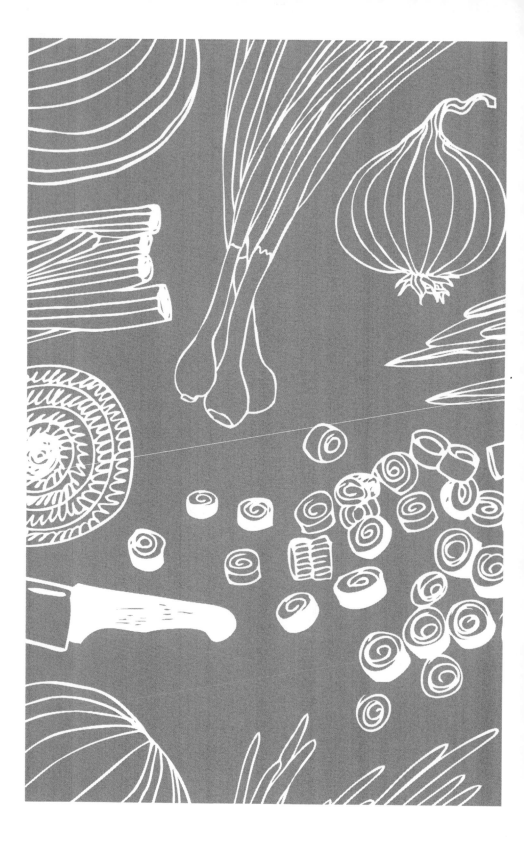

Glossary

Aerobic exercise: Makes your body use large quantities of oxygen, such as running, biking, and swimming.

Agave nectar: A natural sweetener that's about 40 percent sweeter than sucrose (white sugar). Made from the agave cactus, it ranks lower on the glycemic index than other sweeteners.

Amino acids: The building blocks of protein. Your body breaks down protein into amino acids in order to use it.

Antioxidants: Phytonutrients, vitamins, and minerals that protect your body from free radicals to promote good health.

Artificial sweeteners: Laboratory-made substances designed to replace sugar, such as aspartame. Prevalent in diet sodas; not recommended on the Clean Eating plan.

Blood glucose: The form of sugar that's in your blood.

Body mass index (BMI): The proportion of your height to your weight. A healthful BMI is on the lower end of the spectrum—between 18.5 and 24.9, depending on your bone structure and muscle mass.

Calories: The units of measurement of the energy in food. Higher calories mean more energy; if you eat more energy than you use, your body stores it as fat. A calorie from fat contains the same amount of energy as a calorie from carbohydrates.

Carbohydrates: The main food energy source used by your body, found in plants. Carbohydrates are either simple or complex. Simple carbs are broken down by the body quickly and can cause blood sugar fluctuations. Simple carbohydrates have very little nutritional value and include white sugar, honey, and white flour. Complex carbohydrates take longer to digest and are full of fiber, minerals, and vitamins. Healthful complex carb sources include vegetables, fruit, legumes, beans, and grains.

Chia seeds: The chia plant is a member of the mint family and its seeds are highly nutritious. These seeds soak up about nine times their volume in liquid, so they make great thickeners and puddings.

Chlorophyll: This is the green pigment that absorbs the light required to provide energy for the process of photosynthesis in green plants.

Coconut oil: The oil extracted from coconut meat when it's put through a centrifuge. It is thought to have many health benefits including helping to lower cholesterol, boosting the immune system, assisting with weight loss, and promoting proper digestion.

Complete proteins: A protein that contains all nine essential amino acids. Essential amino acids are not produced in the body, so they have to be obtained in food. Dairy, red meat, eggs, poultry, seafood, and fish are all complete proteins.

Diet: Whatever you eat, not necessarily related to a weight-loss or health-improvement plan.

Essential amino acids: The amino acids that your body can't produce at all, or not in the quantities it needs. There are nine essential amino acids, which come from protein or supplements.

Essential fatty acids: These are fats that are essential to the workings in the body. They have to be obtained in food because the body does not produce them. Omega-3 fatty acids and omega-6 essential fatty acids are the most commonly known.

Fiber: Also known as bulk or roughage. This is the part of plants that's not digestible, which means it moves through the body and helps move stool. It can help prevent heart disease, diabetes, digestive issues, and some cancers such as colon cancer.

Flavonoids: Substances found in almost all plants that act as antioxidants in the body, helping to prevent cell damage. There are more than six thousand known flavonoids.

Flaxseed: The seeds from the flax plant. Very high in many nutrients and fiber; a great source of omega-3 fatty acids.

Free radicals: Oxygen or nitrogen molecules that do not have electrons in complete sets. They cause damage in the body because they try to take electrons from surrounding cells to complete the electron set. Too many free radicals can contribute to the development of heart disease, dementia, cancer, and diabetes.

Gluten: A protein that's found mostly in cereal grains. Many people are sensitive to gluten and must avoid all foods containing it.

Glycemic index: A measure of the speed at which your blood sugar levels rise after eating a particular food.

Glycemic load: A measurement that indicates the carbohydrate content of a food based on its glycemic index.

Grass-fed meat: Meat produced from animals that aren't factory-raised, but are raised in pastures and allowed to graze naturally.

Hemp seeds: The seeds from a variety of the cannabis plant. Hemp seeds contain all the essential amino acids, which makes them a great choice for vegetarians. Hemp seeds come hulled or unhulled (which means it's the whole seed with the crunchy outer shell intact). Hulled seeds contain less fiber but are easier for most people to eat.

Insulin: A hormone that helps your body move glucose from your blood into your cells, where it's used for various functions.

Kukicha twig tea: A super food that consists of the stems and stalks of *Camellia sinensi*, a tea shrub. This tea contains six times the amount of calcium as cow's milk, almost three times the vitamin C as oranges, and many vitamins and minerals.

Lactose: A sugar found in milk. For many people it is a digestive irritant and allergen.

Macronutrients: The categories of nutrients that your body uses for essential tasks. They include protein, carbohydrates, and fat and make up the main part of your diet.

Metabolic rate: The rate at which your body uses calories.

Micronutrients: Nutrients such as vitamins and minerals, which your body needs in small quantities.

Omega ratio: The ratio of omega-3 fatty acids to omega-6 fatty acids in food. Ideally, the amount of omega-3 should be higher than or equal to the amount of omega-6.

Omega-3 fatty acid: A group of three fats (ALA, EPA, and DHA) essential for good health and not produced by the body. Omega-3s help cell walls form and assist with almost every cell activity. They are found mostly in fatty fish.

Omega-6 fatty acid: Unsaturated fatty acids, such as linoleic and arachidonic acid, that aren't made by your body but are essential to your health. Omega-6s can help fight cancer and treat diseases like arthritis.

Phytonutrients: Chemical compounds found only in plants. They have many beneficial effects, including cutting the risk of diseases like cancer, cardiovascular disease, and stroke.

Prebiotics: These are the nondigestible carbohydrates that serve as food for probiotics, helping them grow, multiply, and stay in the digestive tract.

Prediabetes: A condition when you have higher-than-normal blood glucose levels; indicates that you're at risk of developing diabetes.

Probiotics: Live bacteria that aid in digestion and help eliminate bad bacteria in your body.

Processed foods: Foods that have been treated with chemicals, preservatives, additives, and dyes. Not recommended on the Clean Eating plan.

Protein: An essential nutrient that your body uses for many functions, including maintaining and building lean muscle mass.

Protein powder: There are three commonly used protein powders: whey, soy, and casein protein, which are commonly available in most supermarkets, health food stores, and online. Whey is a by-product left over after milk is made into cheese. Whey protein is fast-absorbing, which means it's good right after a workout. Soy protein powder is a plant-based protein source and easier to digest than whey or casein. Casein protein is the main protein in milk and is slow-absorbing.

RDA: The recommended daily allowance of food components, such as vitamins and minerals.

SAD: The standard American diet. This diet has all the features that contribute to disease and obesity. It's high in animal fats, processed foods, and hydrogenated fats while low in plant-based foods, fiber, and complex carbohydrates.

Spirulina: A super food that is a form of blue-green algae that grows in freshwater bodies. It can boost the immune system, improve blood pressure, and lower bad cholesterol levels.

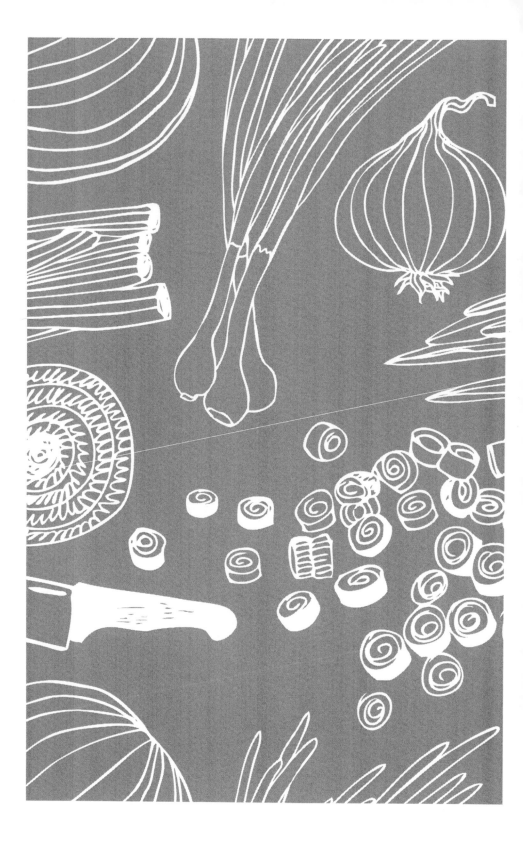

References

BodyandHealth.Canada.com. "High Cholesterol." Accessed July 27, 2012. http://bodyandhealth.canada.com/channel_condition_info_details.asp?disease_id=148&channel_id=41&relation_id=10852

Collins, Sonya. "The Truth about Belly Fat." WebMD. Accessed November 13, 2013. www.webmd.com/diet/features/the-truth-about-belly-fat?page=2.

dLife. "12 Best Fiber Foods." Accessed November 13, 2013. www.dlife.com/dlife_media/diabetes_slideshows/12-best-fiber-foods?index=9.

Ebeling, Catherine, and Mike Geary. "The Top 10 Super-Spices That Protect Your Body." Our Better Health. October 8, 2012. http://ourbetterhealth.org/2012/10/08/the-top-10-super-spices-that-protect-your-body/.

Environmental Working Group. "EWG's 2013 Shopper's Guide to Pesticides in Produce." Accessed November 13, 2013. www.ewg.org/foodnews/summary.php.

Goto, Kazushige, Naokata Ishii, Shuhei Sugihara, Toshitsugu Yoshioka, and Kaoru Takamatsu. "Effects of Resistance Exercise on Lipolysis during Subsequent Submaximal Exercise." *Medicine and Science in Sports and Exercise* 39 (February 2007): 308–15. doi:10.1249/01.mss.0000246992.33482.cb.

Gucciardi, Anthony. "Water with Lemon Each Morning Fights Fat, Boosts Immunity." NaturalSociety. Last modified July 16, 2013. http://naturalsociety.com/water-with-lemon-each-morning-fights-fat-boosts-immunity/.

Harvard School of Public Health Nutrition Source. "Fiber: Start Roughing It!" Accessed November 13, 2013. www.hsph.harvard.edu/nutritionsource/what-should-you-eat/fiber-full-story/.

Hensrud, Donald. "Is Too Little Sleep a Cause of Weight Gain?" Mayo Clinic. April 14, 2012. www.mayoclinic.com/health/sleep-and-weight-gain/ AN02178/.

Hyman, Mark. *The Blood Sugar Solution: The UltraHealthy Program for Losing Weight, Preventing Disease, and Feeling Great Now!* New York: Little, Brown and Company, 2012.

Jacob, Aglaee. "Damaging Effects of Too Much Sugar in the Diet." Healthy Eating. Accessed November 13, 2013. http://healthyeating.sfgate.com/ damaging-effects-much-sugar-diet-1508.html.

Mayo Clinic Staff. "Exercise: 7 Benefits of Regular Physical Activity." Mayo Clinic. Last modified June 23, 2011. www.mayoclinic.com/health/exercise/ HQ01676.

Mckee, Gabriel. *Food Additives.* Chicago: Learning Seed, 2008.

Merali-Ebrahim, Natasha. "Cinnamon—More Than Just a Spice." Just In Time Wellness. Accessed November 14, 2013. http://www.justintimewellness.com/ articles/articles/cinnamon-more_than_just_a_spice!/.

National Cancer Institute. "Cruciferous Vegetables and Cancer Prevention." Last modified June 7, 2012. www.cancer.gov/cancertopics/factsheet/diet/ cruciferous-vegetables.

PsychEducation.org. "Metabolic Syndrome." Last modified February 2003. www.psycheducation.org/hormones/Insulin/metabolic.htm.

Reno, Tosca. *The Eat-Clean Diet: Fast Fat-Loss That Lasts Forever!* Mississauga, ON: Robert Kennedy Publications, 2007.

Roodenburg, Annet J. C., Rianne Leenen, Karin H. van het Hof, Jan A. Weststrate, and Lilian B. M. Tijburg. "Amount of Fat in the Diet Affects Bioavailability of Lutein Esters but Not of Alpha-Carotene, Beta-Carotene, and Vitamin E in Humans." *American Journal of Clinical Nutrition* 71 (May 2000): 1187–93. http://ajcn.nutrition.org/content/71/5/1187.full.pdf+html.

Teicholz, Nina. "What if Bad Fat Is Actually Good for You?" *Men's Health*, October 10, 2007. www.menshealth.com/health/saturated-fat?fullpage=true.

Tomiyama, Janet A., Traci Mann, Danielle Vinas, Jeffrey M. Hunger, Jill DeJager, and Shelley E. Taylor. "Low Calorie Dieting Increases Cortisol." *Psychosomatic Medicine* 72 (May 2010): 357–364. doi:10.1097/PSY.0b013e3181d9523c.

University of Minnesota. "Dietary Ginger May Work against Cancer Growth." *ScienceDaily*, October 29, 2003. www.sciencedaily.com/releases/2003/10/031029064357.htm.

Venuto, Tom. *The Body Fat Solution: 5 Principles for Burning Fat, Building Lean Muscle, Ending Emotional Eating, and Maintaining Your Perfect Weight.* New York: Avery, 2009.

WebMD. "Portion Control and Weight Loss." Last modified May 26, 2012. www.webmd.com/diet/control-portion-size.

Wedro, Benjamin. "High Cholesterol." eMedicineHealth. Last modified February 16, 2012. www.emedicinehealth.com/high_cholesterol/page3_em.htm.

Women Fitness. "Ugly Truths about White Flour." October 2, 2011. www.womenfitness.net/ugly_truths.htm.

Worden, Jeni. "Carbohydrates." NetDoctor. Last modified December 5, 2011. www.netdoctor.co.uk/focus/nutrition/facts/lifestylemanagement/carbohydrates.htm.

Index

Made in the USA
San Bernardino, CA
13 February 2014